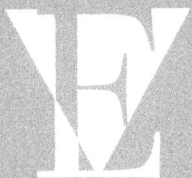

ELITE VOICES

BRAIN RESET

7 STEPS TO A
HEALTHIER BRAIN

BRAIN RESET

7 STEPS TO A
HEALTHIER BRAIN

DR. SPENCER ZIMMERMAN

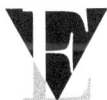

ELITE VOICES

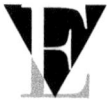

ELITE VOICES
San Antonio, TX 78229

First Edition, October 2023
ISBN: 978-1-63765-496-5
Library of Congress Control Number: 2023917419

Our mission is to empower individuals and businesses to enhance their professional brand by becoming recognized experts in their field. We provide the tools and resources to help our clients become authors, establish a strong personal brand, and grow their business to achieve greater visibility, credibility, and financial success.

CONTENTS

INTRODUCTION
Brain Reset: 7 Steps to a Healthier Brain

Your Amazing Brain

Take a moment to marvel at your brain's tremendous strength. We know that our brain is powerful, and it controls all our body's systems, along with everything else we think or do. But have you ever taken the time to really ponder just what an amazing little machine it is?

Right now, as you read this, your brain is causing your heart to beat and your lungs to breathe, and it's allowing your body to fight against gravity to sit up straight. It's focusing your eyes on these words and rapidly translating what you see into something you can understand. Most amazing of all, it's doing all of this with minimal effort or conscious thought from you.

Every time a new cell phone, computer, or piece of technology is released into the market, we're taken aback by how advanced these products are and by their new capabilities. Yet we take very little time to stand in wonder at the most amazing supercomputer of all—the one that weighs only three pounds and sits on top of our shoulders—our amazing brain.

I've always had an interest in medicine, and I knew that I wanted a career that would enable me to help others. I invested tens of thousands of dollars in school and countless hours studying, yet I found myself sitting listlessly through lecture after lecture. The passion I expected to feel just wasn't there. I had a deep-rooted love for all things scientific, yet most days I felt as if the actual technical aspects of my courses were lacking. I wanted to delve into the mysteries of the human body and the nervous system that controls everything we do, yet none of the professors ever took me to a level deep enough to satisfy my profound curiosity. Everything I learned seemed just to skim the surface.

I needed more.

Feeling completely dejected and wholly unsatisfied, I was about to admit defeat and tell my wife that

I'd wasted much of our savings and gone into considerable debt for nothing. There was no way I could continue with an education that wasn't teaching me anything. My wife is a supportive partner, but there was no way this conversation would go over well. I was consumed with guilt, but I also knew that the rest of my life's happiness depended upon this decision.

Luckily for me, things were about to change.

Right before I was about to trudge home from class and break the bad news to my wife, a fellow student shared with me a video called "Hope Restored" and encouraged me to watch it. That video changed my life, and I wouldn't be where I am today without it. It spoke of a medical approach that provided the answers I'd been looking for. The doctor it featured not only gave hope to the patients he treated, but he filled me with renewed hope as well. I knew I needed to begin my journey into chiropractic/functional neurology.

Immediately my new career choice offered me the knowledge I'd always sought. Ten years later, I can proudly say that I live the life I always dreamed of. I've treated thousands of patients—including NFL, NHL, and UFC athletes, in addition to countless Special Forces soldiers and individuals from all over the world—many of whom were suffering from traumatic brain injuries or concussions. Most were at their wit's end after searching for answers to help heal their injuries and illnesses and relieve their symptoms. I'm grateful I was the one able to help them. Through intensive treatment and therapy, their hopes were restored.

While my professional life was going better than I ever could have expected, someone close to me was suffering in silence. I'd return home from work each evening and recount all the fantastic things I'd seen that day. I'd talk about my patients' symptoms and explain to my wife all the different therapies we implemented. As time passed, she eventually said she'd been dealing with many of those same symptoms but had considered it a normal part of her life. If this was happening to her, how many others were in her same boat?

Because I was still learning, it took a bit of detective work over the course of a few years, but I was finally able to help my wife who was suffering needlessly from the effects of post-concussion syndrome. Diving into her history, I discovered a long list of traumas she'd endured that were never adequately treated. In middle and high school, she suffered two substantial car accidents. When eventually seen by a doctor for the first one, she was treated for minor whiplash symptoms and sent home. A few years later, she was in another accident, and while she was a bit stiff and sore, she did her best to continue her daily life as if nothing had happened.

While she was never aware of any direct trauma to her head or brain, her list of symptoms was telling. She experienced chronic headaches, extreme dizziness (especially when turning), nausea, fatigue, balance issues, and insomnia. Her list of symptoms seemed endless, and my heart went out to her.

On top of all this, we also discovered that she was severely allergic to gluten. Just the smallest amount of it brought on pounding headaches, brain fog, and an upset stomach. She also broke out into strange, pimple-like rashes when she consumed dairy. She needed help, and I was going to do anything I could to give her relief.

That's how the seven steps to a healthier brain were born.

Through this seven-step program, I was able to identify my wife's symptoms and diagnose her issues. Thanks to daily exercises and lifestyle changes, she now leads a much more normal life, and many of the things that once plagued her are gone completely. Her dizzy spells are almost completely gone, and her balance has dramatically improved. She can now go on a run and turn to look over her shoulder without having to come to a complete stop. Her mind no longer races, and she gets both the quality and duration of sleep her body needs to function correctly throughout the day. When I see the energy she has as she races around the backyard with the kids, I know we've made tremendous progress. She's lost the fifty pounds she gained as the result of carrying five children and is the happiest and healthiest she's ever been.

A happier, healthier life can be yours too, and I'm going to show you how.

Throughout this book, we're going to discover just how amazing our brain is. We'll look at how a healthy brain functions and delve into all the symptoms and issues that arise when our brain isn't functioning optimally.

We'll also take a deep dive into the seven most important steps you need to take to keep your brain healthy or to restore function if an injury has occurred. We'll discover the hazards of brain inflammation, what causes it, and what we can do to minimize it. We'll look at the complexities of the nervous system and the connectivity channels in the brain. Plus, we'll uncover all the critical things we can do in our everyday lives to improve the health of our brain—such as eating and sleeping correctly, getting the proper physical activity, and working on brain-based exercises to improve brain connections—and ultimately lead to better brain function.

Emotional well-being is a vital part of our brain health as well. Healing PTSD and emotional trauma is crucial for optimizing our brain function and ultimately living our best possible life.

When you really stop to consider it, the human brain is a funny little thing. It weighs only about three pounds and has the consistency of Jell-O, yet it's one of the most powerful, mysterious things on the planet. Despite this, taking care of our brains is often one of the last things that we think about. Brain health usually only comes up when we begin to suffer the effects of a concussion, traumatic brain injury, or stroke. It also comes up when we suffer from or watch a family member battle memory loss, dementia, or Alzheimer's. If we wait till there's a diagnosis of Alzheimer's or dementia to pay attention to our brain health, it's often too late to have a substantial impact on our condition.

We spend much of our youth worrying about our weight and our diet, focused on how we look. As we get a bit older, we may take our heart health or our metabolic health into consideration. We chase so many different symptoms and bounce from provider to provider, blaming our thyroid, hormones, adrenals, and gut. However, seldom do we ever think about the tiny machine controlling all of it from upstairs.

If you give it some thought, how can any other part of our body function efficiently if the one that orchestrates it all is impaired in any way?

It can't.

This book will change all of that for you. I'll tell you everything you need to know about boosting your brain health in order to function better and increase your vitality—all by healing your amazing brain.

Ready to take a stand? It's time for a brain reset.

"

The implications of an unhealthy brain are far-reaching, and early identification of compromised brain health is vital. Our brain determines not only our potential, but also who we are.

"

CHAPTER 1

7 Steps to a healthier brain

Your Health and Your Brain:
Symptoms and Diagnoses

In the first two chapters, I'll introduce you to the foundational principles upon which everything in this book is built. These chapters are loaded with information and are intended to help you gain a better understanding of what's going on, before taking steps to improve your brain health. When you understand the "why," then the "what to do" will all make sense.

- Chapter 1 dives into common symptoms and diagnoses of a brain that isn't healthy, explaining these concepts in detail.

- Chapter 2 explores what actually occurs in an unhealthy brain and provides insight into why you haven't responded to other treatments. You'll gain an understanding of what aspects of your brain health aren't being addressed so that you can finally start getting answers.

Before you go further in this chapter, if you know your brain is unhealthy and don't care about understanding the why, feel free to skip to the first step in improving your brain health by proceeding to chapter 3.

The Forgotten Organ

When you think about your health, how often do you think about your brain? If you're like most of us, you likely don't consider the health of your brain very often. Even if it's struggling, you might feel nothing can be done, so you continue pressing forward.

During our yearly trips to the doctor's office, the physician checks our pulse and blood pressure. They may check our reflexes, examine our eyes and ears, and run a panel of blood work to determine if there are any deficiencies or abnormalities. Very seldom, however, do they ask us questions or perform any evaluations relating to the health of our brain. The brain is only evaluated after a severe traumatic brain injury or a stroke, or when obvious signs of dementia are present, which is a major problem.

Through millions of lightning-fast electric impulses, our brains work continuously, sending signals that keep us alive and allow us to move, think, and feel. If the health of this vital organ diminishes, so too do many different aspects of our well-being. The implications of an unhealthy brain are far-reaching, and early identification of compromised brain health is vital. Our brain determines not only our potential, but also who we are.

Symptoms of an Unhealthy Brain

Knowing the signs of an unhealthy brain is extremely important. Let's take a look at some of the most common symptoms that could indicate an underlying problem affecting proper brain function.

Brain Fog

"Brain fog" is a term used to describe a foggy or fuzzy feeling. You may feel spaced-out or confused, or as if your brain isn't firing on all cylinders. You may also find it challenging to remain focused and your ability to concentrate diminished. You may find that you have difficulty remembering things, or maybe you're just generally more forgetful than usual.

Dizziness

Feeling faint, woozy, and unsteady are all signs of dizziness. You may experience these symptoms when you move suddenly, or they can be present when you're standing still or lying down. They may also come on as short attacks that last only a few moments or persist for more extended periods. Being dizzy is often described as a shifting, unsteady, or spinning motion. It can leave you feeling weak, nauseous, and anxious.

Word Finding

Have you ever been at a loss for words? The word you needed was right there at the tip of your tongue, but you couldn't verbalize it? The inability to find a specific term when you need it can indicate that parts of your brain aren't connecting appropriately.

Mood Changes

Have you noticed your mood changing lately? Perhaps you're usually a happy, optimistic person, but recently have felt down and depressed for no obvious reason. Nearly all mood disorders are caused by improper connections or inflammation within the brain. Many things can impact these connections, such as head injuries, diet, infections, stress, and traumatic events.

Insomnia

Insomnia is an issue that plagues so many of us. Not being able to fall asleep at night or not getting the quality of rest we need can leave us feeling tired throughout our day. Sleep is a vital part of our day as it's during this time that the body recovers and repairs itself, and the brain removes toxic wastes.

Poor Concentration/Easily Distracted

Do you find it extremely difficult to concentrate, or are you becoming more easily distracted? Maybe you feel you have ADHD. Not being able to focus on one thing for an extended period is an indication that your brain isn't functioning as it should be.

Fatigue

It's entirely normal to feel tired, even exhausted, after a long, busy day. Feeling excessive, ongoing fatigue, however, isn't normal. You may wake up in the morning and still feel extremely tired, as if you hadn't slept at all, or you may have extreme difficulty performing even the most basic tasks. You'll have trouble thinking clearly, and it will be hard to get your body to make simple everyday motions. Individuals routinely blame their thyroid, hormones, and blood sugar for their fatigue, forgetting about the brain, as it weighs only a few pounds and uses about 25 percent of the body's entire energy supply.

Poor Coordination

Having good coordination means that you can move different parts of your body together smoothly and without issue. When poor coordination occurs, you may experience balance issues, dizziness, and feelings of frustration.

Balance and Gait Changes

Balance and gait changes leave you unsteady on your feet. Walking in a straight line becomes difficult, as does maneuvering over any type of uneven terrain. Changes in your balance and gait can make it extremely easy to trip, fall, and injure yourself. Balance and gait are also two of the best indicators that the brain isn't as healthy as it should be, whether due to an acquired injury or a neurodegenerative process in the works.

Short-Term Memory

Our short-term memory is the part of our memory system capable of holding on to information for a relatively short period. Our short-term memory helps get us through our days, allowing us to remember our appointments and schedules, where we parked our car, and where we put our keys. When our brains can't hold on to small pieces of data for short amounts of time, it's a good indication that our health is suffering. [Reminder: We normally lose our long-term memory last, even with dementia.]

Diagnosis Given for an Unhealthy Brain

When one or more of the above symptoms present themselves, it's usually a clear sign that the brain's health is suffering. It's proof that something isn't functioning correctly and has manifested itself in physical symptoms requiring immediate diagnosis and treatment. While many diagnoses may be given, there aren't specific diagnoses for all abnormal connections or processes that may occur. However, we're going to delve into some of the most commonly diagnosed illnesses of the brain.

Developmental Diagnosis

This type of diagnosis often occurs in early childhood after a child's basic learning skills and developmental markers have been examined to determine if they're progressing and learning appropriately. Currently, one in six children experiences some form of developmental delay, and this number is increasing.

These delays can present in the form of behavioral issues, language problems, or difficulty learning. These issues often start during fetal development and progress throughout a person's life. However, some developmental delays can arise due to a traumatic injury or infection during childhood.

As a child grows, they reach specific developmental milestones, such as their first smile, their first wave, and their first steps. Monitoring these milestones is one way to determine whether the child is on track and developing at an appropriate rate for their age. If any delays are noted, a doctor will recommend developmental screening, which will test the child's abilities and provide immediate intervention to help correct any issues that arise.

Some of the most common forms of developmental diagnoses include:

- **Autism**—Also known as autism spectrum disorder (ASD), this condition is characterized by problems with social, emotional, and communication skills. A child who has ASD may:

- Avoid eye contact and want to be left alone

- Repeat the same actions over and over again

- Not point at objects or not have any interest in things shown to them

- Have trouble adapting to changes in their routine

- Exhibit difficulties expressing their needs

- Lose skills they once had

- **ADD/ADHD**—Attention deficit disorder or attention deficit hyperactive disorder is most commonly diagnosed in children. However, it can be discovered in anyone at any age. In the United States alone, it's estimated that between 3 and 5 percent of the population is diagnosed with this disorder. A person who has either ADD or ADHD will show symptoms such as:

  - Poor ability to focus for even short periods

  - Poor organization skills

- Poor memory skills

- Lack of motivation

- Fatigue

- Restlessness or anxiety

- Fits of rage

- Impulsive behavior

- **Dyslexia**—This learning disability is usually diagnosed in school-age children. It's a common condition characterized by an inability to read, write, and spell correctly. People affected by dyslexia will have an average intelligence level and normal vision. Those diagnosed with this condition may:

  - Have difficulty learning and identifying numbers

  - Have difficulty learning and identifying letters

  - Frequently misspell words

  - Have difficulty learning to read

  - Have difficulty learning and participating in school

- **Processing Disorders**—Processing disorders can be broken down into multiple subtypes, such as visual, auditory, and sensory classifications. These disorders occur when the brain has difficulty correctly receiving and responding to information it receives through the senses. Some of the most common symptoms of this disorder include:
    - Difficulty remembering spoken instructions
    - Difficulty focusing if there's an abundance of background noise
    - Difficulty engaging in conversations
    - Difficulty discerning between different shapes or objects
    - Difficulty walking and moving correctly around objects
    - Appearing clumsy
    - Refusing to wear specific clothing because of the way it feels
    - Disliking being touched
    - Using excessive force, even for the smallest of tasks

- Having a strong desire to touch things or people

- Exhibiting extreme behaviors and tantrums

Acquired Injuries

As the name suggests, acquired injuries are those we receive through injury or illness. The most common reasons for an acquired brain injury to occur are as a result of infection, specific diseases, a lack of oxygen to the brain, or direct trauma to the head.

Acquired injuries can be broken down into two main types, nontraumatic and traumatic. The most common types of traumatic injuries are caused by car accidents, falls, sports injuries, recreational activities, physical assault, domestic violence, and explosions.

Depending on the part of the brain damaged, a variety of symptoms may be present. Common symptoms that occur after acquired brain injuries are:

- Headache

- Poor concentration

- Dizziness

- Difficulty sleeping

- Mood changes

- Fuzzy or blurry vision

- Brain fog

- Vomiting or nausea

- Difficulty speaking or finding words

- Chronic fatigue

- Short-term memory loss

Some of the most common forms of acquired brain injury diagnoses include:

- **Concussion/Traumatic Brain Injury—** This type of injury occurs typically after a sudden, forceful impact to the head, body, or whiplash motion. The most common form of traumatic brain injury is a concussion. To suffer a concussion, a loss consciousness isn't necessary.

- **Stroke—**A stroke, also known as a cerebrovascular accident (or CVA), occurs when the blood supply leading to the brain becomes disrupted. This causes a lack of oxygen to the brain and other body areas, often leading to severe and permanent brain damage. Nearly 20 percent of strokes that occur each year happen to someone who previously had one in the past five years.

- **Anoxic Brain Injury**—An anoxic brain injury occurs when the brain is starved of oxygen for an extended period of time. This can occur during birth if the umbilical cord gets wrapped around a baby's neck, or it can happen during strangulation, choking, drowning, anaphylactic allergic reaction, heart attack, or from trauma to the windpipe. Brain damage can begin to occur when the brain has been deprived of oxygen for as little as thirty seconds. The longer the deprivation, the more damage that will occur.

- **Cerebral Palsy**—This condition, known as CP, is a disorder that usually happens at birth or very early on in life. "Cerebral" refers to the brain, while "palsy" means having to do with the muscles. Therefore, this disorder causes a weakness in the muscles because of a problem with the brain.

- **Infections**—A variety of infections and toxins—including COVID, flu, pneumonia, herpes, Lyme disease, and mold—can cause a brain injury.

Degenerative

Degenerative brain conditions occur as we age, but these are happening at younger and younger ages. The underlying process starts ten to twenty years before serious symptoms appear and a diagnosis is given. The key to preventing these conditions from occurring is to stack the deck in your favor and be proactive while you feel good.

With degenerative conditions, the neurons in the brain begin to deteriorate, causing a decline in the brain's ability to function. Degenerative brain conditions usually start very mild and are blamed on other things. They continue to worsen over time, significantly affecting the quality of life and, in many cases, resulting in death. Despite a great deal of research in this area, there is no cure for these diseases. Treatment options have helped slow the progression of these diseases, but as of yet, nothing can stop them. It's essential to recognize early symptoms as it may be possible to prevent the disease from manifesting or delay the onset with early care.

Many things contribute to the progression of degenerative brain conditions, such as toxins in our environment, toxins we put into our body (like alcohol, drugs, cigarettes, and processed foods), chronic stress and anxiety, chronic sleep disorders, blood sugar imbalances, chronic inflammation, head injuries, PTSD, and frequent infections.

Some of the most common forms of degenerative brain diagnoses include:

- **Alzheimer's**—It's estimated that over five million Americans are currently living with some degree of Alzheimer's. This number is expected to triple to nearly fifteen million by 2050. Symptoms of this disease usually begin to appear when a person passes sixty, and it continues to progress steadily from then on. The disease usually begins with mild confusion and forgetfulness, but will further develop to present with the following symptoms:
  - Memory loss
  - Misplacing items
  - Forgetting essential names and places
  - Sleep problems
  - Difficulty speaking
  - Obsessive behavior

- Changes in mood

- Significant weight loss

- Delusions

- Difficulty balancing a checkbook

- Difficulty performing daily routines without assistance

- **Parkinson's**—Parkinson's is a disease that first impacts movement and bowels; it can be very debilitating. There is no known cure for this disease; however, numerous different treatment options can help minimize symptoms and slow down its progression. This disease directly affects the nervous system, causing tremors, muscle stiffness, and difficulty performing movements, including walking. Nearly 70 percent of individuals will also develop a form of dementia. The symptoms of Parkinson's disease consist of:

  - Muscle tremors and shaking

  - Stiff muscles

  - Difficulty with balance

  - Changes in posture

- Difficulty performing automatic movements

- Difficulty speaking

- Difficulty writing

- Constipation

- Loss of smell

- Memory loss

- **Multiple Sclerosis**—Also referred to as MS, this disease affects the central nervous system. It's considered an autoimmune disease in which the body begins to attack itself, breaking down the myelin coating on the body's nerves, causing lesions to form. Because myelin allows for information to be sent quickly, this makes it extremely difficult for the brain to transmit messages throughout the body properly. The most common symptoms of MS include:

  - Numbness or weakness on one side of the body

  - Tingling sensations in the limbs

  - Tremors

- Sensations of electric shocks throughout the body

- Difficulty walking

- Problems with vision

- Fatigue

- Dizziness

- Difficulty speaking

Mental Health Diagnoses

Mental health diseases can occur in anyone at any age and for a wide variety of different reasons. Many are caused by concussions or traumatic brain injuries and may take years to develop after the injury. Some mental health issues are brought on due to hormone and chemical imbalances in the brain, while others are present due to exposure to traumatic events. Some mental health issues may be genetic and are passed down through inheritance. Some problems may occur due to exposure to long-term, chronic stress. While the reasons for mental health diagnoses may vary greatly, one thing remains clear: the brain is responsible for our moods, and an unhealthy brain is sure to result in poor mental health.

Some of the most common mental health diagnoses are:

- **Depression**—Depression affects over 300 million people worldwide, making it one of the most common brain-health diagnoses. This disease is characterized by persistent, long-term feelings of sadness that lead to a loss of interest in once-enjoyable activities. The primary symptoms of depression include:
    - Feelings of sadness
    - Feelings of being unworthy
    - Feelings of guilt or hopelessness
    - Changes in weight and eating habits
    - Extreme fatigue
    - Loss of interest in activities, food, or relationships that previously were enjoyable
    - Sleep disorders
    - Loss of focus and difficulty concentrating
    - Thoughts of death
- **Anxiety**—Anxiety is a feeling of chronic dread, nervousness, or fear of a perceived threat. This feeling of anxiety is usually

unwarranted and can often spiral out of control, leading to decreased quality of life and even panic attacks. It can keep you from doing activities you once enjoyed and can lead to further feelings of depression. The most common symptoms of anxiety include:

- Fear

- Hyperventilation

- Racing heart

- Excessive sweating

- Chest pain

- Shaking

- Headaches

- Cramps

- Difficulty breathing

- Dizziness

- Thoughts of death

- **PTSD**—Post-traumatic stress disorder is a mental health diagnosis caused by a highly stressful, life-threatening, or traumatic event. This event is usually life-altering in some way and leaves the person who experienced it suffering from the aftermath. Symptoms of PTSD include:

- Nightmares

- Hallucinations

- Anxiety

- Depression

- Mood swings

- Difficulty coping during regular activities

- Flashbacks

- Feelings of guilt

- Irritability

- Sleep issues

- Reckless behavior

- Difficulty concentrating

There are many different symptoms and diagnoses that can reveal an unhealthy brain. Much of what we do during daily life affects the health of our brain and, therefore, our overall health and well-being. Actively being aware of any symptoms we're experiencing and any family history of mental illness or brain disorders, and doing everything possible to keep our brains free from trauma and as safe as possible, can go a long way to improving our health.

If any of the symptoms or conditions we've mentioned in this chapter sound familiar to you, don't worry. We'll continue to look into the importance of brain health in the following chapters and take a deep dive into the *7 Steps to a Healthier Brain*.

Summary

- One may experience many symptoms that suggest their brain isn't healthy, including brain fog, fatigue, headaches, and problems with finding words.

- Diagnoses for an unhealthy brain fall into three main categories: neurodevelopmental, acquired injuries, and neurodegenerative.

- Despite having many diagnostic labels, there isn't a diagnosis for everything, and it's most important to understand the underlying process of why the symptoms are there to begin with.

"

We often think about how the
actions we take throughout our
day will impact the health of our
bodies, but rarely do we think of
their direct impact on our brains.

"

CHAPTER 2
The Unhealthy Brain: Understanding What Happens

Our brain determines not only who we are, but also our potential and what we achieve. Whether your goal is to maintain or improve your brain health, understanding this chapter is essential.

I've worked with numerous individuals who went through divorces following a brain injury, as well as with individuals who were never able to contemplate marriage due to developmental disorders. Beyond that, the brain impacts every type of relationship you can have with friends and family, and those you can build at work. Families are ripped apart as a loved one battles dementia.

Your brain determines your ability to excel at work and to have the career of your choice. If you've suffered from brain-based symptoms, you've likely seen your performance drop, or you've been passed over for a raise, or, even worse, you've lost a job.

Maintaining a healthy lifestyle is one of the most important things we can do to enhance our quality of life and increase our longevity. We often think about how the actions we take throughout our day will impact the health of our bodies, but rarely do we think of their direct impact on our brains.

An unhealthy brain can either come from a process that has gone on for decades and has finally manifested, or it happens in an instant from a brain injury.

Americans' number one health concern is dying from dementia. We all know someone who has been impacted by this terrible disease process that starts ten to twenty years before a diagnosis is given. The first symptoms often start with misplacing things and progress to an inability to remember the date, what was eaten the day before, and, even worse, names of family members they've known for years. The question that needs to be answered is whether your brain health will last as long as your body. If the answer is no, then understanding what happens in the unhealthy brain is a must.

We know that an unhealthy brain can lead to a whole host of symptoms, some of which are annoying and uncomfortable, and others that can have significant, detrimental effects on our day-to-day lives. While many different types of brain illnesses can be diagnosed, they all share an underlying dysfunction that can be broken down into four main issues: inflammation, energy crisis, impaired connectivity, and problems with blood flow and oxygen. These factors play a significant role in the brain's overall health, and all four can overlap and influence one another, so we're going to take a detailed look at these main aspects that contribute to an unhealthy brain.

Inflammation

You've probably heard the term "inflammation" before. You've probably said you feel inflamed. It's a term often thrown around in health literature as something we should try to treat and prevent, but the concept can be complicated, and it's often difficult to answer why it's there in the first place. While there are complicated reasons for inflammation, many basic things can cause it, which we'll touch on shortly. It's important to remember that inflammation in the body does not always stay localized and can greatly impact the brain. So what exactly is inflammation?

When you hear the term "inflammation," I want you to think of it as one of the ways the body communicates. Inflammation is a natural response of our immune system. It's entirely normal, helps keep us safe from bacterial and viral attacks, and aids our bodies in recovering from injuries. Think back for a moment to the last time you cut your finger. As soon as this mishap occurred, your body's immune system sent out an army of white blood cells to protect the area from further harm and to initiate the healing process. This caused acute inflammation, causing the area to become red, warm, and swollen. Within a few days, as the cut began to heal, the inflammation subsided, and the repair process began. A very similar process occurs when we become sick. White blood cells wage war on the invading pathogen, fighting it off and keeping our bodies healthy.

While this acute inflammatory response is entirely natural and, in fact, helps keep us alive and healthy, chronic inflammation is altogether a different story. Let's take a step back to the example of getting sick. As the white blood cells are successfully beating the infection, signals are released, letting the body know it doesn't need any more troops for the battle. Chronic inflammation occurs when those signals aren't received, and the response isn't stopped. This causes the body to feel that it's under a constant state of attack, and the immune system shifts into a chronic inflammatory state. Many associate this with an overactive immune system, but that's an oversimplification.

Think of the immune system as a seesaw. Part one is about identifying and killing bad guys, and part two is about allergies, parasites, and stress responses. When part two is persistently present, it creates more fog and confusion in the immune system. It prevents individuals from effectively fighting infections and from shifting back into a state of balance. This can manifest as joint pain, brain fog, problems finding words, and changes in behavior from eating certain foods.

The exact causes of chronic inflammation and the way each individual describes it are different. Regardless, diet, stress, lack of exercise, obesity, poor sleep, concussion, traumatic brain injury (TBI), infections, environmental toxins, heavy metals, and unhealthy lifestyle habits (such as drinking, smoking, and drug abuse) are all contributing factors.

As these factors are left untreated or uncontrolled, this chronic inflammation can rage through the brain and body like a wildfire, and continue to become an ever-increasing problem as we age. This isn't good because our brain's immune system naturally shifts to a more inflammatory state as the years pass, and it doesn't need any extra help heading in the wrong direction. The stress in our lives and the toxins we are exposed to over the years will lead to some level of inflammation in our older years. This inflammation is made worse if you're dealing with head injuries, obesity, hypertension, diabetes, and autoimmune diseases.

Inflammation can also begin before we're born and while we're still going through the early, crucial stages of development. If your mother is in a constant state of stress, enduring chronic infections or making poor lifestyle choices, the inflammatory effect will trickle through to the fetus in utero. These factors may contribute to the rise of autism spectrum and other neurodevelopmental disorders.

Chronic inflammation can affect all areas of the body, including the brain. This is called neuroinflammation and may occur due to any of the factors we've already mentioned, or it can result from a brain injury. When this inflammation occurs, the brain becomes infiltrated with immune cells, and the resident immune cells change, impairing the brain's regular activity. This can lead to developmental disorders such as autism, ADD/ADHD, and processing disorders or cognitive disorders as we age, such as Alzheimer's and dementia. It also plays a major role in recovery from brain injuries and stroke.

By the time Alzheimer's and other dementias are diagnosed, neuroinflammation has been raging for ten to twenty years. Early recognition of this inflammation and prevention of it are the best defenses against these aggressive processes.

With every episode of inflammation, the brain begins to lose neurons, which reduces its capacity and functioning power. This leads to chronic inflammation: immune cells change in the brain and become locked in a state of destruction, instead of shifting to a repair state. Reducing this inflammation and calming down the body's overactive immune response is an essential part of minimizing the damage that chronic inflammation can cause.

Signs of brain inflammation:

- When you get sick, you suffer with headaches, brain fog, forgetfulness, and mood changes.
- When you eat inflammatory foods, you feel foggy, lose words mid-sentence, and lose motivation.
- You feel you're too young to be getting dementia, but always seem to be misplacing objects.
- You make lists so that you won't forget what needs to be done for the day; if

you don't, dinner will start late, or a kid may not be picked up.

- Operating on less than a full night's sleep causes you to drag physically and cognitively, resulting in both reduced job performance and impaired ability to interact with friends or family.

Energy Crisis

Did you know that although our brain makes up only approximately 2 percent of our body's total weight, it uses nearly 25 percent of the body's energy? The mitochondria in our cells are the energy producers. When these cells begin to malfunction, a whole host of developmental and degenerative brain diseases can occur.

As an energy crisis ensues, the brain struggles to perform its regular tasks, using more energy in the process. It becomes an inefficient machine. We take for granted how awesome our brain is and that simple tasks are no longer simple when the brain isn't healthy.

Imagine that a car, which should be able to get thirty miles per gallon, only gets fifteen. This means, when you fill up the tank, the car goes only half as far as it used to. If it goes half as far, then you can accomplish only half of what you could have previously accomplished when it was at its optimal level. The same thing is true for our brain. As the day goes on, symptoms such as headaches, brain fog, forgetfulness, mood changes, and problems finding words may increase.

This inefficiency triggers an immune response and causes increased inflammation in the brain, leading to a vicious circle of even lower energy levels and even higher levels of inflammation. If you have preexisting inflammation, this will also challenge energy production.

Brain injuries, such as concussions, cause an energy deficiency. This is why one of the most common symptoms of a brain injury is chronic fatigue. If you're dealing with chronic fatigue, then you've likely chased your thyroid and hormones, hoping they hold the answers. I find nearly 30 percent of my patients have completely normal thyroid levels, and the cause of their chronic fatigue is an unhealthy brain.

Signs you're suffering from an energy crisis:

- When performing tasks such as reading, responding to emails, or studying, you become tired.
- No matter how much sleep you get, you wake up exhausted and struggle to make it through the day.

- When physically or cognitively exerting yourself, such as when walking, running, reading, or using the computer, you notice cloudy thinking, neck pain, headaches, or mood changes.

Impaired Connectivity

Our brain is formed of billions of neurons connected by synapses. Messages travel at lightning speed from one area of the brain to another via electric impulses through these synapses. The more connections we have in our brain, the faster our brain processing can be; we can think and react to stimuli faster. This supports a process called "neuroplasticity," which is the brain's ability to learn. Plasticity can be positive or negative, depending upon the stimulation and habits formed. We see specific conditions and symptoms with negative plasticity, which we'll discuss shortly. When the brain becomes unhealthy due to inflammation or injury, its functioning ability and connections are significantly reduced.

In developmental conditions of the brain, such as autism, ADHD/ADD, dyslexia, and other processing disorders, there's a problem with the way the brain sends messages: the neurons aren't firing correctly, there's a delay in sending or receiving information, or there's an incorrect connection between parts of the brain. Incorrect connections can become too strong and cause negative beha viors, such as being quick to anger, irritability, and needing a reward to perform a task.

Abnormal connection patterns are commonly seen in PTSD, OCD, and depression. Certain networks should be supported in a healthy brain, but with those symptoms and conditions, it changes. The key to helping those individuals is changing the network connections in a positive direction.

When there's an injury directly to the brain, such as brain injury or stroke, certain connections become broken or damaged, preventing the transmission of specific information. In some cases, these connections can be repaired. However, depending upon the extent of the injury, some are too severe to be fixed, and the goal is to optimize the healthy neurons so that they function at a higher level. This is what happens with strokes and severe traumatic brain injuries.

As mentioned earlier, chronic inflammation also plays a substantial role in the connectivity of the brain. If there's too much inflammation, the synapses won't be able to pass messages between the neurons properly. More simply put, inflammation cuts through the connections in the brain and rips it apart.

While brain-based rehabilitation is awesome and life-changing, the results are short-lived if the causes of inflammation aren't addressed. The destruction of connections is especially seen in cognitive diseases such as Alzheimer's, dementia, autism, and Parkinson's due to unresolved inflammation.

To perpetuate this vicious cycle, the more impaired the neural connections in the brain are, the more inflammation is created; therefore, a bigger energy crisis occurs, which negatively influences connections.

Signs your brain isn't connecting appropriately:

- You forget why you walked into a room or where you placed your keys.
- When reading or writing, you flip letters or numbers and have been referred to as dyslexic.
- When asked questions or trying to retrieve information, it takes you longer to respond, and it feels as if you can't process normally.
- You get upset or irritated quickly without first processing what was said or done, leaving others frustrated with your behavior.

- You're unable to let thoughts go, which negatively impacts your day.

Blood Flow and Oxygen

Sufficient blood flow and oxygenation are imperative for a healthy, well-functioning brain. The brain requires three times more oxygen than our muscles. The blood vessels that supply the brain with blood can narrow and widen as the body needs to ensure that a sufficient supply of nutrients is always available. The brain can survive for only approximately two minutes without oxygen, after which it will begin to die.

The blood also carries a supply of glucose to the brain, which is its primary fuel source. Sufficient glucose in the bloodstream and proper blood flow are imperative for the brain to function correctly and get the energy it needs to work efficiently.

When the blood flow to our brain is compromised, oxygen levels are significantly decreased. We most commonly think of this when a stroke occurs, even though there's a blood-flow reduction following concussions and traumatic brain injuries as well. The areas of the brain that have smaller blood vessels usually suffer the most severe consequences.

An excellent example of decreased oxygenation of the brain occurs when people travel to areas of higher altitudes where oxygen in the atmosphere is lower, which results in less oxygen in the blood as well. Symptoms of altitude illness include headaches, extreme fatigue, loss of appetite, nausea, confusion, brain fog, and in severe cases, shortness of breath and even coma.

Individuals with a concussion, TBI, stroke, dementia, Alzheimer's, Parkinson's, autism, and other anoxic injuries have impaired oxygen and blood flow. They're susceptible to even the most minor changes in blood flow and oxygen levels.

For example, after a concussion or TBI, blood flow and oxygen levels have been found to be reduced for at least a year.

You may have your oxygen concentration measured using a pulse oximeter when you go to the doctor, but this doesn't accurately reflect oxygen levels in the brain. It was discovered that even though levels appeared normal at rest, when performing brain-based tasks, oxygen levels dropped. This explains why symptoms increase with too much cognitive stimulation following a concussion or TBI, and may persist for decades following the injury.

Remember, when blood flow and oxygen are impaired, this negatively impacts brain connections, inflammations, and energy crises. Each of these must be evaluated and addressed, or you'll remain stuck in a chronic, self-perpetuating cycle.

Signs of impaired oxygen and blood flow:

- When you travel to higher altitudes, you notice headaches, problems with word finding, or you feel foggy.
- Your MRI shows small-vessel disease.
- Your labs show anemia due to either an iron or vitamin B deficiency.
- When your blood pressure is too high or low, you have brain fog, headaches, and reduced energy. This can be seen with postural orthostatic tachycardia syndrome (POTS).

The Brain-Body Connection

While it's easy to think of our body as being made up of separate parts, it's important to remember that everything is connected. The health of one area is entirely dependent upon the health of all the others.

I want you to imagine breaking your arm. What happens when it's in the cast? Is it just that part of your arm that gets weaker? No. Everything you would normally use—including your wrist, forearm, and shoulder—will lose muscle strength.

Since our brain is the machine that runs it all, keeping it healthy and functioning at its optimal level is vital to experiencing overall well-being. Stack the deck in your favor, and don't forget about the influence of the brain on your body's health.

You've likely blamed your body for many of your symptoms when your brain was the real culprit. Common symptoms blamed on the body, but which may originate from the brain, are depression, brain fog, headaches, constipation, indigestion, vision changes, and chronic fatigue—hence the brain-body connection and why it isn't possible to reset only one or the other. It's all connected.

Our blood supply is shared by all our body parts. Having a healthy, sufficiently oxygenated, nutrient-rich blood supply is vital to keeping everything functioning as it should. Luckily, we have something called the blood-brain barrier, which works as a highly effective filtration system. This barrier is a semipermeable membrane made up of epithelial cells, and it allows some substances to pass through, while keeping out harmful ones. This blood-brain barrier works to keep the brain healthy by blocking dangerous toxins, and it works well in healthy individuals. However, the brain isn't protected by the blood-brain barrier as it should be in those who have experienced head trauma, developmental disorders, and neurodegenerative disorders, which make the brain susceptible to any number of harmful chemicals, inflammatory compounds, and infections.

It's vitally important to remember that everything we do, everything we eat, and all our lifestyle choices affect not only our entire body but, most importantly, the health of our brain as well. Luckily, we have control over the well-being of our brain and can influence how well it functions. We're incredible beings who can unleash the power the brain naturally possesses to lead us to a happier, healthier life. Our brain is designed to heal itself and prevent permanent disease, but we must first identify why it's suffering. If we're conscious of our actions and how we're feeling, we can alter our brain health. We can take the appropriate steps to improve it.

Summary

- Unhealthy brains have four things in common: inflammation, energy crisis, impaired connectivity, and changes in blood flow and oxygen.

- Inflammation is like a forest fire, and many factors can cause it to burn, including stress, poor sleep, head injuries, strokes, infections, and environmental toxins.

- The ailing brain doesn't produce and use energy as it would when healthy; the result is an energy crisis. Less efficient energy usage results in reduced cognitive and physical functions.

- The brain's wiring sometimes doesn't connect appropriately. Over time, this results in permanently weakened or completely destroyed connections, but it can also result in some areas being hyperconnected. We see changes in connectivity in the brains of those suffering from PTSD and depression.

- Blood flow carries nutrients and immune responses to every part of the brain as well as the body. Reduced blood flow and oxygen levels are seen when the brain isn't healthy due to degenerative, developmental, or acquired changes.

- Don't forget the body is connected as a whole. Things that impact the brain impact the body, and vice versa.

You can achieve anything you're disciplined enough to seek. Commit today to supporting your brain health so that you can live life to your fullest potential.

The next seven chapters will teach you how to start to unleash your potential.

When we're sick, the inflammation created by our condition isn't always localized in the body part affected; it often impacts the brain.

CHAPTER 3
Fighting Inflammation

We took some time in the preceding chapter to talk about inflammation and the dangers it presents to your brain's health. This chapter will take a deeper dive into just how dangerous inflammation can be, what can cause it, and, most importantly, what we can do to minimize it and regain our well-being.

I want to introduce you to Jane, a twenty-five-year-old female who was involved in a car accident and was receiving care for a concussion. After only five days of treatment, she noticed less brain fog and neck pain, and fewer headaches and problems with word finding. Her energy increased, her focus improved, and she processed information faster. She could participate at work and not feel overwhelmed or frustrated because she was no longer struggling. She was excited and ready to take on the world.

Unfortunately, she hit a speed bump in her recovery and was out sick for five days. When she returned to the office, she didn't feel as well as she had previously. Many of the symptoms were creeping back; they weren't as bad as they'd been initially, but they were still a concern. She was frustrated because she didn't know why she regressed.

When we're sick, the inflammation created by our condition isn't always localized in the body part affected; it often impacts the brain. This inflammation rips apart the connections in the brain and impacts how energy is created and utilized. We used targeted nutrition, which we'll talk about later in this chapter, to quiet Jane's inflammation and get her back on track.

If you battle symptoms brought on by head injuries or neurodegenerative or neurodevelopmental disorders, then you've likely noticed something similar.

What Is Inflammation?

Inflammation is the body's natural response to injury, illness, or disease. Acute inflammation usually has a sudden, severe onset and lasts only a few days. This type of inflammation is vital when fighting off illness and injury, and it helps our bodies heal. Acute inflammation fights off viruses and bacteria and promotes healing in injured areas of our body. The body sends out immune cells to fight off invading pathogens and to repair damaged cells.

I want you to imagine a disaster response. I grew up on the Gulf Coast, and after a hurricane blows through, it's time to clean up. Some parts of the damaged houses and buildings need to be completely removed, but others need to be partially removed so rebuilding can occur. The same thing should happen within our immune system, whether it's battling the results from a cut or a brain injury.

Inflammation, however, becomes dangerous when it's long-lasting. Chronic inflammation usually begins with minimal-to-no symptoms that gradually increase in severity over time and can have a severe impact on your quality of life and overall health. This process can take decades and is what we see in nearly all neurodegenerative conditions. The effect of type 2 diabetes on cognition is a great example of unresolved inflammation.

With this unresolved inflammation, specific parts of the immune system go into overdrive, constantly sending out immune cells and specialized chemicals to recruit more immune cells to fight a threat that often doesn't exist. When this occurs, the body can experience a wide range of different symptoms, such as:

- Body aches and pains

- Insomnia

- Constant fatigue

- Depression, anxiety, and other mood disorders

- Gastrointestinal issues, such as diarrhea, constipation, and acid reflux

- Weight gain

- Frequent infection

- Brain fog and difficulty concentrating

- Diagnosis of autoimmunity

- Memory loss or problems with finding words

Inflammation occurs when the body's immune system is triggered. This trigger may be a real threat, such as a pathogen, or it may be a perceived threat that was dealt with, as is the case with some causes of chronic inflammation. Anything that places a long-term stress load on the body—such as diet, stress, blood-sugar imbalance, hormone imbalance, poor sleep, head injury, stroke, or environmental factors—can ignite the process of chronic inflammation.

As the immune system detects the threat within the body, it goes into overdrive, dilating capillaries, increasing blood flow, and sending out an army of white blood cells and leukocytes to fight the invaders. When the bad guys are defeated, signals should be released telling the troops to go home. With chronic inflammation, this doesn't occur.

If there is no virus or bacteria to fight off, the immune system can turn on its own body, attacking organs, tissues, and healthy cells, which can lead to autoimmunity. This creates a shift in the immune system, and a vicious cycle begins. As the body becomes weaker and the cause of this inflammation isn't addressed, the immune system continues to pump out immunity mediators, which in turn adds stress to the body and signals further immune responses, all of which increases inflammation. This circle will continue until the cause of the inflammation is addressed.

Unfortunately, routine lab work doesn't pick up many of the causes of inflammation.

What Is the Blood-Brain Barrier?

Luckily, a healthy brain has a protective layer that keeps it safe from chemicals and pathogens. This layer is made up of tightly packed endothelial cells that act as a filter, allowing nutrients to pass through to nourish the brain while keeping everything harmful out. Think about a well-guarded community. The only way in is through the gate if you're on the list, but unwanted visitors can't get in.

In a healthy, well-functioning brain, this barrier keeps out inflammatory cells and chemicals, protecting the brain from symptoms of inflammation. However, after illness or trauma, the blood-brain barrier can become damaged, putting the brain at risk of further illness and leading to neuroinflammation. Specific injuries—such as stroke, anoxic brain injury, and traumatic brain injuries—routinely lead to an opening in the blood-brain barrier.

With neurodegenerative conditions, the barrier has been breached and remains open years before a diagnosis is ever made.

What Is Neuroinflammation?

Neuroinflammation is inflammation of the nervous system's tissue, and it can occur in certain parts of the brain or the brain as a whole. Many psychological disorders are thought to be directly related to neuro-inflammation, as are neurologic and somatic illnesses like Alzheimer's and Parkinson's. When this occurs, the neurons of the brain become damaged, and the brain's immune cells (microglia) eat the neurons instead of repairing them. This leads to premature loss of neurons, and the brain begins to degenerate, causing a decrease in brain function, which has a negative effect on the entire central nervous system. Common symptoms of neuroinflammation include chronic fatigue, brain fog, difficulty concentrating, inability to handle stimulation in crowded or noisy areas, memory issues, and depression. New studies are also linking this condition with diseases such as type 2 diabetes and heart disease.

Diagnoses associated with neuroinflammation:

- Alzheimer's
- Parkinson's
- Multiple sclerosis
- Traumatic brain injury
- Stroke
- Anoxic brain injury
- Autism
- Concussion
- PANS/PANDAS
- Lewy body dementia
- Depression

This is just a sample list. There are many more.

The Most Common Causes of Inflammation

Chronic inflammation has been linked to many auto-immune diseases, such as Hashimoto's thyroiditis, rheumatoid arthritis, psoriasis, multiple sclerosis, systemic lupus, and possibly chronic fatigue syndrome. While the causes of chronic inflammation are still being studied to better understand how they influence different diseases and injuries, many factors are known to play a significant role in causing it. For most individuals, it's a mix of the factors below, and that's why improving brain health is so hard on your own—you're unaware of the full scope of what's keeping you stuck.

- **Diet**

  A healthy diet is one of the most important factors for maintaining overall good health. A diet that consists of processed food, artificial sweeteners, added chemicals, pesticides, and saturated fats can put undue stress on the body and lead to high levels of inflammation.

- **Chronic and acute infections**

  When the body is constantly trying to fight off attacks from viruses, parasites, and bacteria, the immune system becomes fatigued. This can lead to chronic inflammation and a buildup of toxins. Chronic infections are believed to be the most common cause of autoimmunity.

- **Mold and water-damaged buildings**

  Exposure to mold or bacterial toxins from water-damaged buildings can be highly hazardous to the body. Mold releases microscopic spores that contain mycotoxins, which, with long-term exposure, trigger an immune response and lead to inflammation. Mold is a very common toxin, despite the fact that most people are completely unaware that it impacts individuals in all areas of the world.

- **Traumatic brain injuries**

  While the initial brain injury itself can cause acute inflammation, it may also lead to a state of chronic neuroinflammation that can persist for years. Initially, after the injury the blood-brain barrier is compromised. For some individuals, and due to a variety of causes, the blood-brain barrier subsequently may not close, and a slow but steady destruction occurs to the neurons of the brain, leading to a state of neuro-inflammation. If you had preexisting inflammation before the injury, then this accelerates the process and can keep you stuck in a state of neuroinflammation that will lead to more damage and cell death.

- **Stroke**

    Following a stroke, there is an immediate immune response that creates massive inflammation and opens the blood-brain barrier. However, as is often the case with inflammation, it can quickly spiral out of control, causing more brain-tissue death, which leads to even more inflammation. This is why the state of your health before a stroke occurs is essential to your outcome after it.

- **Gut-brain axis**

    The "gut-brain axis" is a term given to the communication between the central nervous system and the gastrointestinal tract. Our gut contains a multitude of good bacteria and intestinal flora that play a vital role in the functioning of our immune system. When our micro-biota are out of balance, our immune system can't function properly or deal with infection efficiently. It will send bad signals to the brain, and our brain will respond with bad signals in return. This imbalance can quickly lead to chronic and uncontrolled inflammation.

Supplementation Strategie for Reducing Inflammation

While a lifestyle that includes regular physical activity, stress-management techniques, and a healthy diet is important for managing chronic inflammation, many different herbal supplements have also been shown to have a positive effect on breaking the vicious cycle of chronic brain and body inflammation.

Resveratrol

This natural compound is produced by numerous plants, which produce this polyphenol as a defense mechanism to protect them from bacteria, fungi, and diseases. High levels of resveratrol can be found in the skin of grapes, blueberries, raspberries, mulberries, and peanuts. Resveratrol may help lower blood sugar, reduce inflammation, protect the brain, and offer anti-cancer properties. Research suggests it also offers benefits to those struggling with diabetes, Alzheimer's, strokes, and autoimmunity.

Curcumin

Curcumin is the main active ingredient in turmeric. It's one of the most popular spice supplements due to its antioxidant and anti-inflammatory properties. It may benefit those who have suffered a traumatic brain injury or a stroke, and those with multiple sclerosis and even dementia.

Lion's Mane

This interesting mushroom grows long hairlike structures that resemble the shaggy mane of a lion. Studies have shown that lion's mane helps boost brain health by stimulating growth factors that allow brain cells to build connections. These powerful little mushrooms also help reduce oxidative stress in the body, contain numerous antioxidant compounds, and are extremely effective at reducing inflammation throughout the body.

CBD

CBD is an active ingredient found in the hemp plant, a close cousin of the marijuana plant. It contains cannabinoids that have no psychoactive effects on the body but instead have been shown to have significant healing properties. Our bodies have cannabinoid receptors, which are a major area of focus in the research. Studies have shown that CBD can provide pain relief, suppress an overactive immune system, and help reduce inflammation, both systemically and topically. It may also help with sleep, PTSD, and headaches. CBD is available as a tincture, an oral capsule, and a topical solution.

DHA/EPA Fish Oils

Docosahexaenoic acid and eicosapentaenoic acid are omega-3 fatty acids found primarily in cold-water fish and marine algae. They are unsaturated fats that the body requires for proper functioning and that are extremely difficult for the body itself to produce. Supplementing with DHA and EPA is the best way to guarantee that you're getting all the omega-3 your body requires. DHA has been shown to provide substantial anti-inflammatory effects and to also have a positive impact on brain and central nervous system development and cognitive functioning. EPA has a greater impact on body inflammation, blood sugar, and cardiovascular health.

Reishi Mushroom

There is some evidence to show that the reishi mushroom can help positively stimulate the immune system, making it effective in fighting some diseases and cancer. It also has strong anti-inflammatory and detoxifying properties.

Glutathione

Glutathione is made from the amino acids glycine, cysteine, and glutamic acid. While our bodies can naturally produce this substance in the liver, studies have shown that supplementing with glutathione can have a positive effect on our overall health. One reason is that once we pass the age of forty, its levels naturally reduce in our body, creating a negative shift in our immune system. It's also the body's most natural and powerful antioxidant. What exactly does that mean? Well, it grabs inflammatory chemicals or products floating around in the body and takes them out with the trash to lower the inflammatory load in the body.

Astaxanthin

Astaxanthin is a carotenoid found in certain plants, animals, and algae. It has a bright-red color, and its ability to fight free radicals in the body has been shown to be over 6,000 times higher than that of vitamin C. This supplement has a long list of benefits, including strong antioxidant properties, the ability to combat inflammation, brain-health-boosting properties, and an overall ability to fight numerous diseases.

Quercetin

Quercetin is a flavonoid found in many different plant sources. Red wine, onions, apples, grapes, green tea, and berries are known to be high in quercetin. The high levels of antioxidants in this compound make it an excellent immune booster, helping to fight off pathogens and free radicals in the system. It's also been shown to help ease pain and has a significant ability to fight chronic inflammation.

Alpha-lipoic acid

Alpha-lipoic acid is an essential nutrient that the body requires to function properly. Foods such as yeast, broccoli, spinach, potatoes, and organ meat are exceptionally high in alpha-lipoic acid. This fatty acid is best known for its antioxidant properties, but it also plays a significant role in the conversion of enzymes into energy, which takes place in the mitochondria of our cells. Alpha-lipoic acid plays a significant role in the health of our heart and brain, helps manage our blood-sugar levels and weight, and decreases overall inflammation throughout the entire body.

All these supplements may have benefits for both brain- and body-based symptoms and conditions. Symptoms I routinely see improved by them:

- Fatigue
- Brain fog

- Headaches
- Depression
- Insomnia
- Forgetfulness
- Focus
- Blood sugar

The key is finding the right ones for your specific needs and taking a therapeutic dose. The more inflammation you have, the stronger dose you'll need to help fight it. To get the best results, it's best to seek expert help.

It's evident that chronic inflammation, especially when endured long term, can be extremely hazardous to our body's well-being and our brain's health. Many different factors can bring on chronic inflammation, including lifestyle and environmental contributors, as well as traumatic injury to the brain. While some instances of inflammation may be unavoidable, we can take steps to reduce our risk factors for inflammation or increase our ability to recover from it. Leading a healthy lifestyle filled with a nutritious diet and ample physical activity and avoiding toxins can give us the upper hand in stopping inflammation before it starts. Supplementing with a variety of different herbs and dietary additives known to boost our immunity, enhance our brain health, and reduce the amount of inflammation in our body can also help.

Summary

- Acute inflammation is a natural, expected part of the healing process.

- When acute inflammation persists, this is not only highly damaging to the body, but it also takes a toll on the brain.

- Symptoms of chronic inflammation may not appear initially, but will over time.

- Controlling chronic inflammation will make or break brain health more than nearly any other factor.

- There are many causes of chronic inflammation, including head injuries, processed foods, lack of sleep, blood sugar, and more.

- There are natural supplements that may help fight chronic inflammation, including glutathione, DHA, alpha-lipoic acid, CBD, and many more.

"

Think of your brain as a large factory. If this factory doesn't have enough staff to run it, it's impossible to run at maximum output capacity.

"

CHAPTER 4
Supporting Energy and Connectivity

Energy and Our Brain

Think back to the last time you hit the gym or got in an excellent workout. Your legs may have felt wobbly afterward, and your entire body probably felt tired and overworked. The following day you likely woke up with some muscle stiffness and minor muscle aches that resolved themselves over the next day or two. When our brains become tired, however, it's an entirely different thing.

Brain fatigue is very different from body fatigue. When our body is tired, our brain still functions properly; however, when our brain lacks sufficient energy, the symptoms can manifest themselves in multiple different ways, and nothing works the same. You may have difficulty focusing on specific tasks and suddenly feel you have ADD/ADHD. You may find yourself misplacing your car keys or unable to recall what you did last week, which could make you feel your memory isn't as sharp. It's okay. Before we realized my wife was suffering from chronic concussion symptoms, she would leave her phone in the fridge.

When talking with friends, you may forget what you were going to say or have trouble finding the right words to express yourself, even though they were right on the tip of your tongue. You may also begin to experience issues with your moods, becoming easily angered or frustrated. You may even have difficulty sleeping at night. Beyond brain- and mental-health-related symptoms, you may notice that physical symptoms such as constipation, poor coordination, or impaired walking are worse.

Depending upon the cause of this brain fatigue, the resulting symptoms may last anywhere from a few hours to a few days, or even longer. Remember that any of the factors that cause inflammation will worsen brain fatigue.

Our brains are relatively small organs that weigh little more than a few pounds, but they constantly work and control everything that goes on throughout our entire body. Because of this, they are always guzzling fuel and require an enormous amount of energy to continue to function at their optimal level. You've likely taken for granted how much energy the brain uses to perform a simple task such as sending a text or email, reading a book, or interacting with a group of friends.

The brain's primary energy source comes from the perfect combination of glucose and oxygen, which are supplied through the bloodstream. When the nerve cells are active, they require a more significant amount of energy and send signals to the surrounding blood vessels, telling them to dilate in order to release more blood and fuel. This process works exceptionally well; however, in a brain that's suffered some sort of damage or didn't develop properly—either from physical injury or due to disease—blood supply may be limited. This means that the brain's energy source will be restricted, which reduces the brain's capacity to function.

Think of your brain as a large factory. If this factory doesn't have enough staff to run it, it's impossible to run at maximum output capacity. As a result, productivity will be reduced to a fraction of what it should be. Production will focus on the company's most essential parts, and the smaller departments will suffer from the lack of staff.

In our brain, the weakest parts aren't going to get the resources necessary to perform, as energy and nutrients will be shuttled to the most important areas of the brain. Unfortunately, you've likely noticed this. You may not agree on what's most important, but to the brain, it's survival—keeping the body alive. Conscious thought and movement will become secondary to keeping the heart pumping and the lungs breathing. This is why you've experienced forgetfulness, mood changes, poor concentration, and losing your words mid-sentence.

Isn't it an awful feeling when your brain stops making proper connections?

What Is Brain Connectivity?

Think of your brain as a bustling city. There are roads crisscrossing in every direction and cars traveling at warp speed over these roads, bringing messages to and from all the city's inhabitants.

Now imagine the wrong route is taken. What happens? You don't get to your desired destination. This wastes time as you try to get back on track.

The brain is no different. Our nervous system is made up of a multitude of neurons, synapses, and fiber pathways, all of which play a vital role in how the brain communicates with itself and other areas of the body.

This intricate electrical-impulse and data-transfer system moves very quickly and requires a significant amount of energy to operate properly. While we're born with a certain level of connectivity, its level is minimal when compared to the amount needed in order to function properly.

Unfortunately, sometimes the wires get crossed in the brain. We see this with autism, dyslexia, and processing disorders. We can also see injuries to the brain from a concussion, TBI, stroke, or anoxic injury that tears apart these connections. Lastly, degenerative conditions slowly weaken these pathways over decades before a diagnosis is given.

These connections are the result of what is called "plasticity," which is the brain's ability to learn and connect. We learn positive and negative things, depending upon our environment. Have you ever bribed your kid to clean their room, rewarding them with a cookie? Now they want a cookie every time they clean their room, whether you asked them to do it or not, right? That's what we'd call negative plasticity. Our brain is also influenced by internal and external environments.

It's a good thing that it's possible, with some effort, to exercise our brains and create an even stronger level of connectivity. The brain is similar to a muscle that gets stronger the more it's worked. When we continue to learn new things, challenge ourselves with new ideas, and work on making new habits, we can create even more neural pathways, thereby increasing our brain connectivity.

On the other hand, when our brain lacks energy because it isn't getting the proper amount of fuel, creating new connections is virtually impossible. In fact, we can begin to lose the links we already have. (This is already happening anyways—we don't need the extra help.)

As our neural connections become impaired, we can begin to feel the effects of our weakened brain. Symptoms such as memory issues and the inability to focus can persist. Luckily, when caught early enough, we can reinforce these connections and our overall brain function. Since our brains are like a muscle, with some work we can reverse the damage and work toward creating a stronger, more energy-efficient brain, leading to improved energy production.

Dietary Strategies to Support Brain Energy and Connectivity

The food we eat directly determines the quality and efficiency of the fuel our bodies have to use. Imagine for a moment that you own a very expensive, elaborate race car. To get this car to perform at top speeds, you have to fuel it with premium gasoline; anything less could damage the engine. Your body works in the same way. If you fuel it with anything less than high-quality fuel, its performance is going to suffer.

Every time you take a bite of food, instead of focusing on its taste, quickly think about how well it will provide energy for your body. Highly processed foods, such as those from fast-food restaurants or frozen dinners, contain excessive amounts of chemicals, preservatives, and other additives, and have been so extensively processed that very few nutrients remain. They may taste good, but they aren't good for you.

Instead, try and include as many brightly colored fruits and vegetables as possible in your daily meal plan. The brighter the colors, the more vitamins and minerals they contain. Try to choose meat that's been raised without the use of antibiotics, and wherever possible, purchase food that's organic and GMO-free. Healthy fats from avocados, nuts, and fatty fish, like salmon and mackerel, provide omega-3 fatty acids that can provide the brain with extra energy and improve its overall function.

You may be thinking you can eat your way to better health. While that used to be the case, our food supply isn't as full of nutrition as it used to be. This is where targeted nutritional supplements play a role.

Supplements

There are numerous supplements that can help boost your brain's energy supply and enhance its connectivity. Some of the most beneficial supplements for brain health include:

CoQ10—Also known as ubiquinone, CoQ10 is a natural antioxidant that's synthesized by the brain and is vital for energy production. The mitochondria, the energy producers in our cells, pull it in and convert it into a usable energy source. Since our brain contains a higher number of mitochondria than anywhere else in the body, CoQ10 plays an important role in keeping the brain fueled and healthy. CoQ10 is also a powerful antioxidant that protects cells from the damage of free radicals. When we lack CoQ10, we can feel substantial brain fog and forgetfulness, as well as an inability to focus, learn new things, or complete basic tasks.

Acetyl-L-carnitine—This amino acid can be found in animal products and is also produced by the liver and kidneys. The cells of the body use acetyl-L-carnitine to convert fat into a usable energy source for proper brain functions. Studies have shown that supplementing with acetyl-L-carnitine can help improve memory function and may help slow down the progression of some memory-related diseases such as Alzheimer's.

D-ribose—This sugar-like substance is vital to the body's production of ATP (adenosine triphosphate), the mitochondria's main source of fuel. The liver, adrenal glands, and fatty tissue all produce some level of D-ribose, but depending on the body's overall health, the level of available D-ribose may be lacking. Supplementing with this substance can help give the body extra fuel. Studies have also shown that D-ribose has a positive effect on the heart and cardiovascular health, enhancing blood flow and oxygenation throughout the body. This means that the brain will receive better blood flow and, therefore, more energy as well.

Ashwagandha—Ashwagandha is an adaptogen that helps the body respond to stressful situations. An adaptogen is a substance that supports the adrenal glands in a way that is beneficial to the body. It's been shown to reduce the harmful effects of stress hormones (like cortisol) in the brain, promoting healthy brain function and improving energy production.

Lion's Mane—Lion's mane is a specific type of mushroom that is beneficial to cognitive health. One way it does that is through the increase of a growth protein known as brain-derived neurotrophic factor.

Bacopa—Bacopa is a plant that's been used for centuries to help those with cognitive impairment and brain-health issues. While its efficacy is still undergoing scientific study, Bacopa is thought to help protect brain cells from free radical damage and enhance overall connectivity and cognitive function.

Ginkgo Biloba—A powerful antioxidant, ginkgo biloba helps protect the body's cells from oxidative damage. It's also rich in flavonoids that offer added protection to the body's cells, help improve blood flow and energy efficiency in the brain, and may protect against age-related brain diseases such as dementia and Alzheimer's.

Vinpocetine—Vinpocetine is thought to play a significant role in boosting brain health and helping to reverse the effects of memory loss and other brain-related diseases and injury.

Huperzine—Shown to increase the levels of acetyl-choline, Huperzine is a neurotransmitter found in the brain. An enhanced supply of acetylcholine helps improve both the speed and accuracy of neural transmission and can improve energy usage in the brain.

Dihexa (Medical Peptide)—Derived from angiotensin IV, this nootropic drug is known as a peptide hormone. Because of its excellent ability to penetrate the blood-brain barrier, dihexa can profoundly affect the central nervous system and the synaptic connectivity in the brain. It's been shown to create new neural pathways and to help repair those connections that have been damaged. It also aids in the production of mood-related hormones, like serotonin and dopamine, and can slow or possibly even reverse symptoms of dementia-related diseases.

Summary

- Healthy brains produce and use energy efficiently; unfortunately, unhealthy brains do the opposite.

- Start with focusing on nutrition intake to support energy. Excessive carbohydrates usually have a detrimental effect on glucose uptake and negatively impact brain health.

- There are many nutritional supplements that may positively impact energy: acetyl-L-carnitine, D-ribose, CoQ10, and many others.

—— **"** ——

There's actually a direct correlation
between the feel-good hormones
produced in the brain and
the foods we eat.

—— **"** ——

CHAPTER 5
Nourishing Our Brains

I magine you're the proud owner of a new fancy sports car. You spend all your spare time washing and waxing it and driving around town with the top down, showing it off to all your neighbors. You've worked hard and saved every extra penny to make this purchase.

Now imagine driving your new car to the local gas station and getting out to fill up the tank. Which gasoline do you choose? Regular gasoline is the cheapest option, but you know that fueling up with premium gas will be best for the engine and will keep the car purring like a kitten for years to come. I'm sure most of you wouldn't hesitate to splurge and spend a bit more money to give your investment the care it deserves.

While most of us wouldn't hesitate to take extra care of our cars, the majority of society pays very little attention to the fuel we put into our most important vehicle—our bodies.

The food we eat plays one of the most important roles in the health of our body and mind, and it determines the quality of fuel we have to power our brains. All the vital vitamins and minerals we need to not only survive but thrive are found within the foods we eat, and the better the quality of food, the healthier we'll be. Our brains are powerful machines capable of amazing things, but their capacity is limited by how well they're taken care of. It's time to stop limiting your potential and to become all you were meant to be by providing your brain and body with the nutrition they need to flourish. You deserve it.

The Food Paradigm

Unfortunately, we live in a society in which food has become a commodity. No longer viewed as something that must be farmed and produced to keep us healthy, it's instead looked upon by businesses and corporations as a way to make money. Flashy commercials and brightly colored packaging have taken over, and the value of a food isn't based on its nutritional content but on how good it tastes. Instead of picking fruits and vegetables from the garden, food is made on factory assembly lines and from ingredients we can't pronounce. It's pumped full of chemicals and preservatives to extend its shelf life in order to make the most money possible. People in business profit from our food purchases while our health continues to suffer.

Metabolic diseases are on the rise, and obesity is commonplace. Many of us pull into the drive-through multiple times a day and fill ourselves with food lacking even the most basic nutrients. As you dig into your fast-food hamburger, consider for a moment where that meat came from—if it's even meat. You may picture a field of cows grazing on fresh grass and clover. This is what cattle are meant to eat, and meat from free-range livestock contains high levels of protein, amino acids, essential fatty acids, and other nutritious properties. Unfortunately, this beef is also more expensive and would drive the price of our fast food through the roof, making it unaffordable for most.

Instead, the drive-through industry has found a way to acquire their meat cheaply. Feeding cows corn, something their bodies aren't well equipped to digest, can fatten them up quickly. They are then pumped full of growth hormones and antibiotics and forced to live out their short lives in small, uncomfortable pens. If the animals we consume aren't healthy and haven't been appropriately nourished, how can we expect to receive proper nourishment from them?

Another interesting thing to consider is how society views our mealtimes. It's become standard practice among the majority of households to have three very specific meals a day. On top of this strict regimen, these meals must consist of particular foods. Commercials have conditioned us to believe that cereal or toaster waffles are the right thing to have for breakfast, and we shouldn't worry about not getting any fruits or vegetables in the morning because these boxed goods have been fortified with all the synthetic vitamins and minerals our bodies need. We've been conditioned to eat what we're told to eat at the expense of our own health, while companies and agricultural organizations get rich.

We also use food as a way to celebrate. In fact, many people have such a strong emotional attachment to food that binge eating and eating disorders have become highly prevalent. Birthdays, holidays, after-work events, parties, and almost every other occasion center around food, and in most of these cases, the foods that are served are indulgent. We're expected to feast on high-calorie, high-fat dishes and sweet treats; thus, we associate these delicious foods with feeling happy.

There's actually a direct correlation between the feel-good hormones produced in the brain and the foods we eat. There's a reason that so many foods are referred to as "comfort foods": not only are they satisfying to eat, but they also boost levels of serotonin, oxytocin, dopamine, and other endorphins in the brain. Food companies pay scientists an enormous amount of money to make the food stimulate our addiction centers so that we feel deprived without them. These foods literally make us feel happier and reduce our feelings of stress and anxiety—or that's what they want us to believe.

You've likely experienced the crash and withdrawal when trying to clean up your diet. Anything truly good for us shouldn't create such a negative reaction when we're trying to make a positive change. While it's important to feel happy when you eat foods, there shouldn't be a health trade-off that keeps you on a path to hypertension, depression, diabetes, cancer, heart disease, and Alzheimer's. It becomes an issue when we use food as a crutch to make us momentarily feel better when we're down.

The Calorie Myth

It's hard to even think about food without thinking about calories. They're the first thing you see on a nutrition label, and many diet sodas are quick to point out they don't have any. Every new diet fad bombards us with information about calories in and calories out, but do we even really understand what a calorie is? Let's take a minute to break it down.

A calorie is a unit of energy, and one calorie is the amount of energy required to raise the heat of one kilogram of water by one degree Celsius. The more calories that a specific food has, the more energy it contains. If our body doesn't use up the energy we consume, it will store it away as fat for future use. Think about that for a second: all fat is a stored form of energy that needs to be released.

The tricky thing about calories, however, is that not all calories are created equal. Did you know that two Oreo cookies have nearly the same number of calories as two pounds of broccoli? Not only do these two food items differ in physical weight, but they also differ substantially in nutritional value. You would never think cookies are good for you, but you will likely—and gladly—eat them, even though you'd be much fuller and receive many more vitamins and minerals from consuming broccoli.

When you consider which types of foods you're going to eat, focus less on the calories (or even the quantity of food you'll consume), and focus more on the quality of the food. Fresh fruits, vegetables, and free-range meats contain more nutrients and fewer calories than any processed food; therefore, they give your body both the right amount and the proper quality of energy it requires to function optimally. When eating appropriately, you won't consume too many calories because the makeup of your food intake won't allow it. Even better—you won't have to count calories.

Following in Our Ancestors' Footsteps

Take a moment to think back to your ancestors who lived 1,000 years ago. What would they have eaten? Where would they have sourced their food? How would it have been cooked and prepared? The easiest answer to all these questions is straight from nature. The majority of their diet would have consisted of berries, fresh fruits, and vegetables handpicked by them and their family. This fresh produce would have been locally grown and natural for the region where they lived. None of it would have been sprayed with pesticides or would have traveled hundreds or even thousands of miles in a truck.

They would have gotten their protein from wild-caught fish or wild game, or from the few animals they would have raised on their small family farms. Everything they consumed would have been locally grown in the climate where they lived and would have been fresh and virtually unprocessed.

Now imagine attempting to eat like this today. Imagine all the nutrition you would receive from your food. Eating local food not only has a profound effect on the environment, but it can also greatly impact your health. It reduces the need for preservatives and added chemicals to keep food fresh, and the level of vitamins remains higher when foods are consumed at their ripest. In fact, studies have shown that the nutritional value of fruits and vegetables begins to decline in as few as twenty-four hours after being picked. This doesn't take into account that, depending on the part of the country where they're grown, foods have drastically different nutrition profiles.

Unfortunately, the decrease in nutritional value of food over the past one hundred years has created a need for nutritional supplements. This isn't an excuse to avoid fresh foods; foods that are fresh are more flavorful and much more satisfying.

Intermittent Fasting

Besides eating local fresh food, your ancestors would have also practiced intermittent fasting. Mealtimes would have been sporadic and based on the availability of the food. Since food had to be hunted and gathered, it could take hours or even days to kill and prepare the meat, and the search for berries or wild produce could have led them miles away from home. Because of this, their bodies adapted to periods of fasting when they had to survive on their bodies' energy stores for fuel. This is why our bodies have different ways to produce energy.

In contrast, many of us don't ever go longer than the six to eight hours that we are sleeping without eating. When we constantly bombard our bodies with food, we never give them the time they need to take a break from digestion. Intermittent fasting has been used for centuries in many different cultures and religions. It can help to purify and remove wastes and toxins from the body.

Studies have also shown that fasting can have the following benefits:

- It helps balance hormone levels.
- It gives the body time to focus on cellular repair and regeneration.
- It increases the metabolic rate and focuses on burning fat stores for fuel.
- It lowers the level of inflammation in the body.
- It speeds up the growth of new nerve cells and improves brain function.

For most who intermittently fast, there's a window of fourteen to eighteen hours in which food isn't consumed. Normally breakfast is skipped, and the only meals are lunch and dinner.

[Pro tip: If you can, eat breakfast and lunch, but skip dinner for the best results.]

Finding the "Perfect" Diet

A quick search online will bombard you with flashy new diet fads and crazy techniques to lose weight, get in shape, and become healthier. The important thing to remember is that most of the things you read online about dieting are an attempt to make money.

Whether it's the low-fat craze, the keto phase, or any other diet trend sweeping the streets, nothing is as simple and healthy for your body as eating wholesome, clean, nutritious foods, all in moderation and based on your energy expenditure levels. Because we're genetically different, individuals will respond to the same food differently. This is why some individuals do fantastic with a certain diet, while someone else struggles and becomes worse.

We can't emphasize enough the importance of staying away from any diet trends that you may be enticed to try. While many of these diets may have immediate health benefits, they aren't sustainable for long periods of time—meaning that your weight will fluctuate, and your overall health will suffer.

The Dangers of Pesticidesand Other Chemicals

When choosing to eat healthier, most people assume that opting for fresh fruits and vegetables is all that it takes. Unfortunately, this is only partly true. Much of the produce we eat has been sprayed with pesticides to help control the effects of insects, rodents, weeds, fungus, mold, and bacteria that could harm the crop. These pesticides are highly toxic when ingested; the affect our hormone levels, cause autism and ADHD, and even lead to some cancers.

When purchasing your produce, buy local organic produce whenever possible. Growing your own vegetables is another excellent option to reduce your pesticide exposure. Certain foods are known to contain higher levels of pesticides than others. They are known as the Dirty Dozen, as published by the Environmental Working Group on a yearly basis. These foods include:

- Strawberries
- Spinach
- Kale
- Nectarines
- Apples
- Grapes
- Peaches

- Cherries
- Pears
- Tomatoes
- Celery
- Potatoes

If you choose to include these foods in your diet, be sure they're organic and well washed or peeled before eating them.

The lowest levels of pesticides are found in a list of foods called the Clean 15, which include:

- Avocados
- Sweet corn
- Pineapples
- Onions
- Papayas
- Sweet peas (frozen)
- Eggplants
- Asparagus
- Cauliflower
- Cantaloupes
- Broccoli
- Mushrooms

- Cabbage
- Honeydew melons
- Kiwis

Unfortunately, chemicals aren't only found in the produce we eat. There are also high levels of growth hormones and antibiotics found in the meat and dairy products we consume. Animals are pumped full of these harmful substances to enable them to grow at faster rates, produce more milk, and remain free from illness, which leads to increased profits for the farmers. Studies have shown that certain types of cancer, hormone disorders, and earlier puberty rates have been linked to exposure to these substances, but the extent to which these chemicals are detrimental is still being studied. The question you need to ask yourself is if you should take that risk.

Staying Hydrated

Staying hydrated is vital to the health of our bodies and our brains. So many people don't drink the required amount of fluids on a daily basis, which leaves them dehydrated. Don't count soda, alcohol, or juice as part of your fluid intake as they don't really help with dehydration and usually make it worse. When you're dehydrated, your mood can be affected, and you can suffer from headaches and concentration issues. This is because the neurons in your brain fire at a faster rate when there's sufficient fluid to help transmit their messages. This means that you'll be able to think more clearly, act faster, and have more energy to push through your busy day.

When choosing what to drink, clean, filtered water is always the best choice. This contains the fewest chemicals and is precisely what your body requires for optimal hydration. Tap water contains pharmaceuticals, toxins, and metals that aren't properly eliminated. Also, stay away from sugary beverages and those with added caffeine. And, remember, diet drinks are even worse due to artificial sweeteners that your body has no clue how to use. You should drink anywhere from two to three liters (sixty-seven to one hundred ounces) of water per day to achieve optimal hydration, so drink up!

Making the Change

You may feel overwhelmed by the information in this chapter, but don't worry. You can change your diet and eating habits. It's about the direction in which you're moving and building momentum. Do better today than you did yesterday, and you'll get there. In fact, making these changes, bit by bit, will enable you to incorporate them into your daily life in a way that provides confidence and is maintainable for the long term. This means that you'll be more likely to stick with them and reap the benefits of a healthy diet for the rest of your life.

- Fast—Practice intermittent fasting by eliminating the first meal of the day and striving for a fasting period of fourteen to eighteen hours. For example, if you finish dinner at 7:00 p.m., don't have another meal until 12:00 p.m. If you do this, you will have fasted for seventeen hours. It's okay if that's too much initially, but I know you can work up to this. Start by doing this once a week to give your body its much-needed break, and slowly incorporate this fasting into your daily routine.

- Balance your meals—Imagine that a plate in front of you is divided into three different-sized sections. The largest section should be overflowing with an abundance of vegetables. The second-largest should contain your proteins and fats, and the smallest section should contain healthy carbohydrates such as berries or (occasionally) gluten-free grains. Now, every time you sit down to eat, make sure that your plate is laid out this way!

- Eat the rainbow—When you pick your vegetables, strive for a wide variety of types and colors. These will all have different but vital nutrients that your body needs for optimal health. Vary your meals with a combination of both raw and cooked vegetables, eating as much raw as you can to get the highest level of nutrients possible. If you're unable to eat raw, then try steamed as the next option, with panfrying being the worst choice.

- Pick the best quality meat—If you choose to include meat in your diet, make sure it's organic and has been raised and fed properly, without the use of antibiotics or steroids. Organic, grass-fed beef is a good choice, or opt for wild game when possible. When consuming fish, make sure that it's wild-caught and not farmed, and completely avoid tilapia. Salmon, mackerel, and other wild-caught fish are loaded with essential fatty acids, which are excellent for our brains.

- Watch your carbs—Try to avoid grains whenever possible, specifically those that contain gluten. Most people can't digest gluten well, and it can lead to a number of different health problems. When consuming carbohydrates, focus on eating a wide variety of different berries that have been grown organically without the use of pesticides. Other fruits are fine to incorporate, but try to eat only those that are local and in season, and avoid eating too many high-sugar fruits like watermelons, mangos, and pineapples.

- Healthy fats—In addition to wild-caught fish and grass-fed beef, there are other sources of fat. If you're trying to lose weight, it's good not to continually have these though. Consider instead walnuts, pecans, almonds, coconut butter, almond butter, olive oil, avocados, and eggs.

- Season your food—Use a wide variety of different seasonings to enhance the flavor and nutritional value of your food. Choose fresh herbs and spices, but try to stay away from added salt or highly processed flavorings.

- Try prebiotic and fermented foods— Prebiotic and fermented foods contain healthy bacteria that are important for our gut health and that help boost our immunity. Foods like kimchi, sauerkraut, kefir, kombucha, miso, tempeh, and organic yogurt are all excellent for the health of your gut's microbiome and, therefore, your entire body.

- Stay hydrated—Don't forget to drink between two and three liters of water every day. You can spruce up your water by adding different herbs, fruits, or vegetables; just be sure to stay away from carbonated beverages, alcohol, and fruit juices.

When you begin making these changes, try focusing on just one area at a time. Slowly reduce the amount of food you consume, and when you eat, spend more time chewing and enjoying your food to be sure that it's properly broken down to have the best digestive experience possible and reduce heartburn or indigestion.

Plan out your trip to the grocery store, and spend the majority of your time in the outer aisle, where all the healthiest and freshest foods are kept. Take time when preparing your food, and remember that mealtimes should be a time for laughter and rejuvenating your body.

Summary

When in doubt, do your best to keep these dietary rules in the front of your mind:

1. Eat fresh, locally grown foods.

2. Eat food that is in season.

3. Avoid processed foods.

4. Avoid added sugars.

5. Eat the rainbow.

6. Fuel your body to fuel your mind!

One important thing to always remember is just because a food is considered healthy doesn't mean you couldn't respond negatively to it. For example, don't force yourself to eat avocados or berries if you develop bloating, brain fog, or a skin breakout when you do.

"

During sleep, our brain stores
memories for safekeeping, our
recall ability is improved, and our
mood is boosted, allowing us to be
ready to take on the day ahead.

"

CHAPTER 6
The Importance of Sleep

W e all know that sleep is important, but how often do we trade it to watch a movie, hang out with friends, or go to a concert? Should we sacrifice it so readily? We often think that we can make it up later, but that isn't true. Our bodies and our brains literally can't function without it! Throughout the course of our lives, we spend nearly one-third of our time sleeping. Think about that: if you live to be ninety years old, then you spent thirty years sleeping. Yet humans are the only mammals that voluntarily give up sleep.

Unfortunately for so many of us, our quality and quantity of sleep are lacking. Admit it: you've probably told yourself that you can function just fine with five or six hours of sleep. Although we spend a lot of time worrying about our health and focusing on getting enough exercise, eating a nutritious diet, and making regular trips to the doctor and dentist, few of us take the time to make sleep a priority.

Sleep is one of the most important pillars of our health. It's a time for healing and rejuvenation within the body, and the brain is even more sensitive to lack of sleep. During the hours when we're at rest, the brain goes to work removing toxic waste from the body's tissues, essentially cleaning out the body and tidying up so that we can function at the highest level possible.

Why Is Sleep So Important?

Why do we require sleep every night, and what happens to our bodies if we don't get enough? When we head to bed at night, our bodies start producing hormones that help get us ready for sleep. Melatonin, for example, is released and tells our body it's time to prepare for bed. But melatonin does much more than help us sleep; it plays a role in our immune system's health as well.

Our breathing slows and deepens, our body temperature and blood pressure drop, and our heart rate begins to slow down. Throughout the night, we go through different stages and depths of sleep, and during these stages, our muscles relax, and the blood supply to them increases. When this happens, the body begins its repair cycle; tissues repair themselves, and new muscles, tissues, and cells are created. Our energy levels are restored, and our immune system is rejuvenated, making us less prone to future illnesses and better able to fight off the bacteria and viruses we come in contact with.

Have you ever noticed that when you have a run of poor sleep, you're more likely to get sick, feel foggy, or have an autoimmune flare-up? You may have also noticed that when you're sick, you seem to sleep a lot more.

A good night's sleep is essential to the proper functioning of our bodies and our brains for good overall health. Certain hormones are released during sleep that help us grow and generate new cells, and other growth factors and neurotransmitters are released that tell our brain cells to connect. During sleep, our brain stores memories for safekeeping, our recall ability is improved, and our mood is boosted, allowing us to be ready to take on the day ahead.

Without consistently getting sufficient sleep, we're unable to function properly in our daily lives. Our attention span and concentration levels will be lacking, and we'll be more susceptible to sickness and disease, not to mention overall feelings of lethargy and low energy. Our overall health will be diminished, and we'll be put at much higher risk for a wide variety of different diseases. When we're exhausted from poor sleeping habits, we're more likely to engage in other habits that are detrimental to our health, and we can become stuck in a vicious cycle. For example, you may notice you're much more likely to hit the sofa and spend your spare time being lazy since you just don't have the energy for anything else.

A word of caution...

I get it. You may have gone years with less-than-optimal sleep and haven't noticed any issues. Brain problems such as dementia start twenty to thirty years before a diagnosis. Think of lack of sleep as a slow leak that initially doesn't impact anything, but over time creates massive damage.

> *[One more note: If you're trying to recover from a brain injury, then getting sleep is essential. In my experience, those who struggle with sleep have a very challenging recovery, even if everything else is done correctly.]*

Positive Effects of Sleep on Health

If feeling well rested, alert, and full of energy aren't enough reasons to get a good night's sleep, here are a few more benefits that getting sufficient rest can provide:

- Improved mental health—combatting depression, anxiety, and irritability
- Ability to stay on task at home or work
- Store and retrieve memories, such as family vacations or special events
- Strengthen immune system to be resilient against infections
- Elimination of toxins, specifically within the brain
- Rebalancing hormones, such as testosterone, progesterone, and estrogen
- Regeneration and repair of both body and brain tissue
- Regulation of metabolism, helping to maintain a healthy weight, evening out blood-sugar levels, and boosting cardiovascular health

Everything operates better within the body when sleep is a priority.

What Happens When You Lack Healthy Sleep?

Now that you can see how important sleep is and all the benefits it can provide, it should be easy to imagine all the health hazards of consistently restless nights. There are too many to fully list, but here are some to consider:

- Your memory is no longer as sharp as it should be, and finding words is a challenge.

- You feel as if you were a squirrel and can't stay on task. If you don't complete it at that moment, you may not come back to it.

- Your immune system doesn't get to take care of the bad guys, resulting in risk of infection, autoimmune flare-ups, and chronic inflammation.

- You don't have the energy to engage in life and create memories with your family and friends.

What Is the Circadian Rhythm?

You've probably heard the term "circadian rhythm" before, but do you understand what this concept means and how important it is to your health? Our circadian rhythm is the sleep-wake cycle that governs our days and nights and is controlled by a clock in our brain.

Some individuals function better going to sleep around nine, while for others it may be ten or even midnight. No matter which one you are, the basic principles are that we should sleep for around seven to nine hours.

The circadian rhythm is a master clock that runs on a twenty-four-hour system and dictates which biological activity should occur at what specific time. Triggered by environmental stimuli (like the rising and setting sun), the brain sends signals to synchronize when specific activities should occur within the body. Certain tasks, like tissue regeneration and the storage of memories, are best done while our body is at rest. Other tasks, such as digestion, function best during daylight and are hindered as the clock shifts to night.

If this vital rhythm gets out of whack, it can lead to a whole host of issues, including many different sleep disorders.

Sleep Disorders

A sleep disorder is a chronic condition that causes someone to consistently encounter issues while sleeping. Research has shown that nearly 20 percent of those who have suffered some type of traumatic brain injury, including concussions, will develop a sleep disorder of some kind. Sleep disorders also play a major role in the development of Parkinson's disease.

Insomnia

Insomnia is one of the most common sleep diagnoses. Insomnia is best characterized by the inability to fall asleep or to stay asleep for extended periods of time. Often this is caused by racing thoughts that keep your mind active, even though you feel extremely tired. Even after you fall asleep, you're plagued by restlessness as these thoughts haunt your dreams as well, leading to feelings of exhaustion the following day.

When you're given this diagnosis, you'll likely first try different over-the-counter medications for help, but you may ultimately end up on prescription sleep medications. Unfortunately, these medications hurt the brain when used routinely and can contribute to cognitive decline.

Sleep Apnea

Sleep apnea is a disorder that affects people's breathing patterns while they sleep and causes them to stop breathing for a short amount of time. The pathways to the lungs aren't open fully; therefore, their body and brain don't receive enough oxygen during the night. In more remote areas of the brain, where blood flow is already limited, sleep apnea can be extremely detrimental.

This lack of oxygen means some areas of the brain will significantly lack proper oxygenation. Anyone with sleep apnea will notice symptoms related to this. Because these momentary breathing episodes disrupt the standard sleep patterns, the person's sleep is interrupted; therefore, fatigue and exhaustion often set in during the day. This increases the person's need for sleep, and they may notice they need naps or energy drinks to function.

Sleep apnea can be a dangerous condition. It's very harmful to the brain and cardiovascular system. It's also known to contribute to Alzheimer's and other forms of dementia, as it literally causes the brain to shrink in size at a significant rate. It also makes it very difficult to improve brain health for those who have suffered concussions or developmental disorders.

Treatment for sleep apnea is often aimed at losing weight, as obesity is a very common cause of sleep apnea. For some, this isn't sufficient, though, as many people with normal weight also have sleep apnea. Traditional care involves using a CPAP machine to help get increased air flow, and therefore oxygen, into the body. If the machine is truly needed, it's essential that it's used. Even though it's uncomfortable, it's better to be uncomfortable than to have dementia.

If sleep apnea is minor, some individuals find considerable benefits by using mouth tape and no longer need a CPAP. Mouth tape basically promotes breathing through the nose and reduces the obstruction that creates sleep apnea.

Finding the Right Amount of Sleep for You

Some people can get away with very little sleep and still function efficiently throughout their day, while others need a lot of sleep in order to function at all. Why is this? What's the reason that different people require a different amount of sleep to feel their best?

The answer comes down to genetic expression and cellular function. Our genes and cells are influenced by our environment and dictate our initial circadian rhythm (the wake-and-sleep cycle our body follows). Remember, the environment plays a massive role in this, and it can change your sleep cycle, making it hard to get back to an acceptable pattern of sleep.

Our body releases hormones based on this schedule. These hormones—including thyroid, testosterone, estrogen, progesterone, and other growth hormones—determine what time we get tired and how much sleep we require to wake up and feel rested and rejuvenated.

Most people require eight hours to feel their best, but depending on the person's genes and how active their lifestyle is, it can range anywhere from seven to nine hours. Even if you think you function well on five or six hours of sleep, this will usually come back to haunt you as you age. The longer you wait in life to change your sleep cycle, the harder it is.

If you're unsure how much sleep is right for you, try this experiment: Count backward nine hours from your usual wake-up time, and use this as your bedtime for one week. You may not fall asleep right away, and that's okay. We all need to get off the hamster wheel of life and give our brains and bodies a chance to heal and recover.

For example, if you wake up at 7:00 a.m., make sure that you're tucked comfortably into bed by 10:00 p.m. Make this your regular bedtime for one week, and see if by the end of the week, you're waking up before your alarm goes off. If you wake up thirty minutes to an hour before your alarm goes off, don't try and fight to get back to sleep. Instead, get out of bed, start being productive, and receive exposure to sunlight if it's out. You may find that you need thirty minutes more or less to hit your optimal amount of sleep.

Naturally Improve Your Sleep

If you suffer from poor sleep, here are some suggestions that will help you get a better night's rest every night. They're easy to implement, and once you turn them into a regular routine, you should find that your sleep quality quickly improves, and you have more stamina and focus throughout your day.

If you have had a stroke or are suffering from a brain injury or neurodegeneration, these are principles to build upon as you'll need to improve your brain health as well.

Tips to help with sleep:

- Avoid alcohol after dinner, as it impacts quality of sleep and recovery.
- Exercise in the morning or afternoon.
- Get sun exposure in the morning to start the day off right and signal to your brain the rhythm you want.
- Turn off electronics one to two hours before bed.
- Avoid things that feed your negative emotions, such as news, finances, and difficult decisions.
- Have a consistent bedtime and wake-up time. The more you modify these times, the harder it will be to get good sleep.

- Wear amber lenses one to two hours before bed.
- Soak in Epsom salts, and then go to bed.
- Finish dinner three to four hours before going to sleep, and eat more protein and fat, as compared to carbohydrates, as blood-sugar dysregulation significantly impacts sleep quality.

Nutritional supplements for sleep:

- Chamomile tea
- Melatonin
- Valerian root
- CBD
- Phosphatidylserine

I understand that not everyone will be able to sleep well with these tips, but the less medication, the better. There are no medications that truly promote all the proper stages of sleep without trade-offs.

Improving Sleep Is Possible—It's about Habits.

Don't underestimate the importance of sleep for your day-to-day health as well as your future health. It's easy to put sleep on the back burner and say you'll catch up on it later.

Always ask yourself if the choices you're making are moving you toward the future health you want. If they're not, identify what you can change. Start with one thing at a time, and remember it's about doing something sustainable.

Summary

Sleep is one of the most important aspects of good brain health, but it's also the one thing we routinely give up.

Sleep helps with:

- Cognitive health
- Mood
- Energy
- Tissue repair
- Immune function

"

Just as your muscles need to be continuously exercised to see the best benefits, the brain connects better as a result of regular exercise.

"

CHAPTER 7
How to Exercise for Your Brain

Exercise is the topic that either excites you or instantly makes you roll your eyes. We all know exercise is important, but we're often quick to search for any excuse not to do it.

When we look back over the last thousands of years, our lives have changed drastically. Things have become much more automated, we're able to shop with the click of a button, and a lot of us even work from home. With all these changes making our lives undoubtedly a lot easier, finding ways to include exercise in our daily routines has become an afterthought for many of us.

If we think about our ancestors, they easily incorporated exercise into their daily lives without giving it any thought, simply because they didn't really have a choice. They had to hunt and gather, often walking incredible distances in the span of one day, literally embodying the term "survival of the fittest." Those who were most fit could travel farther to hunt for food and provide for their families because they were more agile. Ultimately, those who were fittest were the ones to survive and pass down their genes.

Nowadays, the most exercise a lot of us get is the walk from our front door to the car, from the car to the grocery store, maybe walking the dog around the block. We spend hours sitting in front of screens, consuming media, and finding the easiest ways to accomplish daily tasks. In order to lead a healthy lifestyle these days, we really have to plan and prioritize our physical activity as there are countless distractions.

When we consider exercising, many of us think predominantly of our physical appearance, losing weight, and building muscle; sometimes we might think about our health or protecting our hearts. However, a lot of us aren't aware of the impact that regular exercise can have on our brain health. Exercise is one of the most transformative things we can do for our brains right now, and nothing can make up for the lack of it.

We've discussed in previous chapters what constitutes an unhealthy brain and how diet can influence brain health. Throughout this chapter, we'll expand upon all the ways in which exercise is paramount for our brain health.

Effects of Exercise on the Brain

We all know that exercise can help us grow muscles, improve our heart health, and even help us lose weight. But did you know that exercise can also improve our cognitive functions, mental health, and memory, while simultaneously reducing stress, anxiety, and depression?

Exercise has endless benefits for the human body. Implementing regular exercise in our routines has also proven to reduce the risk of many types of disease, such as obesity, diabetes, stroke, heart disease, and many types of cancer. In addition, exercise is one of the best ways to accelerate recovery from a brain injury, and it slows or reduces our risk of developing certain neurological conditions such as Alzheimer's and other types of dementia. It does this by protecting the structure and function of our brain as we age. Exercise can improve mood, energy, memory, attention, and focus.

The effects of exercise on the brain are both immediate and long-lasting. Immediately, we see increased levels of dopamine, serotonin, and noradrenaline neurotransmitters. High levels of these neurotransmitters in the brain have been proven to increase our focus and reaction time for at least two hours following a workout. Over the long term, we notice increased brain size, decreased inflammation, and improved mood.

The benefits to brain health attained through exercise all come down to neurogenesis and neuroplasticity. This is accomplished through many ways, but one of the most important is through the release of a growth factor called brain-derived neurotrophic factor (BDNF).

Neurogenesis: "Neurogenesis" is the process in which new neurons are formed in the brain. New neurons are formed during our embryonic stage, as well as throughout our life span, enabling the brain to repair itself and respond to damage or injury. The part of the brain that sees this the most is the hippocampus, which is responsible for learning and memory. Neurogenesis is essential to preventing neurodegenerative diseases.

Neuroplasticity: "Neuroplasticity" describes the brain's ability to change and adapt as a result of stimulation or lack thereof. Through this process, the brain can modify its connections or rewire itself. This is how the brain is able to change as we age; you truly can teach an old dog new tricks. Neuroplasticity also explains how we're able to learn new skills, store memories and information, and recover after a traumatic brain injury or stroke, even if it's been years since the injury.

For a moment, let's consider the brain a muscle. In order to grow our muscles, we focus on targeted exercises. If we want to grow our biceps, we'll do biceps curls. If we want to grow our glutes, we'll do squats. Just as your muscles need to be continuously exercised to see the best benefits, the brain connects better as a result of regular exercise. The parts of your brain that will connect and benefit from exercise are primarily the prefrontal cortex, hippocampus, and cerebellum.

Prefrontal Cortex: Located at the front of your brain, just behind your forehead, the prefrontal cortex plays a key role in executive function; it's the part of the brain that enables us to focus our attention, control emotions, plan, organize, and prioritize. Basically, this part of our brain helps us get through our daily tasks with ease. This is why you notice improved mood and concentration after exercising.

Hippocampus: Located in the temporal lobes, the hippocampus is critical to our ability to learn and to our short-term memory. It is this part of the brain that's routinely impacted by Alzheimer's. Exercise will support neurogenesis in the hippocampus.

These two parts of our brain are the most susceptible to neurodegenerative diseases and normal cognitive decline in aging. By strengthening these parts of our brain, we increase our brain's resistance to degenerative conditions that may impact us.

Maintaining a Healthy Brain

In chapter 2, we covered the four factors that constitute an unhealthy brain: inflammation, energy crisis, impaired connectivity, and blood flow and oxygen. Luckily for us, we can manage these issues through exercise.

Inflammation: We've gone over the negative effects of neuroinflammation and how it can lead to developmental and degenerative brain disorders. Thankfully, we can combat this inflammation in the brain through exercise. Exercise has been shown to alter the activity of the brain's immune cells, in turn lowering inflammation in the brain.

Energy Crisis: As we know, without adequate energy, the brain has a hard time performing its regular, basic tasks. Exercise increases our heart rate and gets blood and oxygen circulating throughout the body. This supports the mitochondria in energy production, enabling the brain to function better and use energy more efficiently.

Impaired Connectivity: Regular exercise benefits the brain through both neurogenesis, which generates and creates new neurons, and neuroplasticity, which is the brain's ability to regenerate itself. Growth factors such as BNDF (brain-derived neurotrophic factor) are released during exercise, and they tell brain cells to connect. Increased plasticity enables the brain to recover quickly after disorders and injuries, and reduces the effects of neurological illnesses.

Blood Flow and Oxygen: Exercise helps circulate blood throughout the body, including the brain, which helps transport nutrients and oxygen to the brain. This increased blood flow enables the brain to perform key functions.

Clearly, we can see the benefits of exercise and how it helps us resist the progression of illness and keep our brains healthy. All the ways that we've discussed in which the brain can become unhealthy are interconnected. When one of these key factors starts to fail, it affects the others and creates a downward spiral. In order to maintain a healthy brain, we must consider all factors individually, but also as a group.

Brain Aging

Aging is an inevitable part of life. As we age, our bodies change, and we become more susceptible to all sorts of illnesses and ailments. Our physical capabilities and cognitive functions gradually decrease. Depending on our lifestyle, we can either increase or decrease our likelihood of developing certain diseases by building up health reserves. This applies to the brain as well.

With age comes a lot of life experience and wisdom, and although we're unable to control our biological age, we can find ways to control our brain age. As our brain ages, certain parts of the brain shrink, communication between neurons becomes less effective, blood flow in the brain decreases, and inflammation occurs. By finding ways to support our brain health, however, we can decrease our brain age, making our brains younger, which enables us to prevent or delay the onset of brain diseases such as Alzheimer's, dementia, and Parkinson's. While the incidence of these diseases is rising rapidly, I strongly believe we can stack the deck in our favor and minimize our risk.

As we age physically, we should incorporate physical activity into our lives to help slow down the inevitable loss of brain volume. This will help prevent memory loss that comes with old age and will lower the risk of degenerative diseases. By decreasing our brain age, we can improve our memory, as well as our ability to multitask and make executive decisions.

Reducing Stress

Our lives are becoming increasingly busy. Most of us spend more time during the week working or worrying about work than we spend relaxing or unwinding. The cost of living is increasing, and some folks find themselves stressed about how to make ends meet. Everything is incredibly fast-paced, and we're always ready for the next thing.

Stress is incredibly damaging to all parts of the body, causing strain that can lead to a plethora of serious health problems, such as heart disease, high blood pressure, and diabetes, among others. In the brain, the stress hormone known as cortisol damages the part of the brain involved in memory and complex thinking. To alleviate this stress, we might turn to anything that will help us shut our brains down, including mindless activities to pass the time and help us forget our problems.

In reality, there's a very simple fix. Participating in some sort of physical exercise throughout the day can have a huge impact on our stress levels and how our bodies respond to stress chemicals. Of course, exercise won't pay the bills or complete the project we've been trying to finish at work. It will, however, reduce our stress indirectly and enable us to function at a higher rate, thereby enabling us to make more money and perform at a higher level.

When we exercise our bodies, we release a bunch of mood-boosting hormones, neurotransmitters, and endorphins, while simultaneously decreasing the number of stress hormones. The hormones released with exercise are as follows:

- **Brain-derived neurotrophic factor (BDNF)**: Released in the brain during exercise, BDNF, a protein, helps promote the survival of nerve cells by playing a role in the growth, maturation/differentiation, and maintenance of these cells, as well as increasing brain plasticity. It's also been suggested that increasing BDNF may lower the risk of depression.

- **Serotonin**: Considered a mood stabilizer, serotonin is a key hormone that increases feelings of well-being and happiness. It's also known to help with sleeping, eating, and digestion.

- **Norepinephrine**: Norepinephrine can act as both a neurotransmitter and a hormone. When acting as a neurotransmitter, it increases alertness and speeds up reaction time. It increases heart rate, blood flow, and energy levels.

- **Dopamine**: Dopamine, a neurotransmitter, plays a role in how we feel pleasure. Increased levels of dopamine can lead to feelings of euphoria, bliss, and increased motivation and concentration. Dopamine is hijacked by mindless activities, including social media, scrolling on the internet, watching the news, and more.

The release of these hormones and neurotransmitters through exercise can help us manage stress and quickly improve our mood. At the same time, we decrease the amount of the following stress hormones in the brain:

- **Cortisol**: Cortisol is important to many functions in our body, including controlling blood sugar, regulating metabolism, controlling blood pressure, and helping the body respond to stress or danger. However, at sustained high levels, this stress hormone can wreak havoc on our body's natural processes. Prolonged high levels of cortisol can lead to inflammation, mental health problems such as anxiety and depression, and health issues like weight gain and heart disease.

- **Adrenaline**: While playing an important role in our fight-or-flight response to fear or a perceived threat, adrenaline speeds up our heartbeat, increases blood pressure, and basically prepares us to react more quickly to a specific stimulus. Despite helping us in moments of panic, increased amounts of adrenaline over an extended period of time can damage blood vessels, increase blood pressure, and elevate our risk of heart attack or stroke. Additionally, it may cause anxiety, weight gain, headaches, and insomnia.

As you can see, exercise is incredibly effective in reducing stress. Balancing these hormones and neurotransmitters in the brain is key to reducing stress. Ultimately, reducing stress through regular exercise will prevent a whole slew of potential future health problems. Because stress presents itself differently in each individual, you may find that suddenly you're sleeping better, no longer have headaches, or have an easier time concentrating after beginning a regular exercise regimen.

Types of Exercise

You might be wondering which type of exercise is the best for our brain health. The answer to that question isn't so simple. The goal with all exercise is to get our heart pumping. That said, any exercise you're committed to doing and find enjoyable is the best type of exercise for you. This will vary for each individual, but the goal is just to get our bodies moving and our hearts pumping. If you know that you have bad knees and you can't run, obviously this won't be the exercise for you, but many low-impact exercises will be just as beneficial to your brain. If you have dementia, it's best to exercise less than thirty minutes at a time as some research suggests increased amounts of exercise can do more harm than good due to increased inflammation.

We can participate in all sorts of exercises to help our brain health. Some of these include, but aren't limited to, the following:

- **Cardio**: Defined as any type of exercise that gets your heart rate up and keeps it elevated for an extended period of time, cardio is known to be beneficial for weight loss and increased stamina. It can reduce the risk of heart disease, high blood pressure, high cholesterol, diabetes, and some forms of cancer. Cardio increases blood circulation throughout the body, which we know helps reduce inflammation and increase energy and brain function. Additionally, it can help with memory and depression, as well as increase our metabolism. Many types of exercise are considered cardio and can be done at home or at the gym: hiking, running, biking, elliptical trainers, rowing, burpees, and dancing are all cardio exercises.

- **Yoga**: Yoga is incredibly beneficial for both the body and mind. This relaxing, meditative exercise helps increase flexibility and balance, strengthen and tone muscles, reduce the risk of injury, increase bone density, and calm the nervous system. Yoga is one of the best exercises for managing stress and anxiety. The various poses and focus on breathing techniques relieve tension, and they can help alleviate pain, sharpen concentration, and eliminate brain fog.

- **Resistance training**: Also referred to as weight training, resistance training is any form of exercise in which you lift or pull against resistance. These exercises can be done with your body weight, free weights, resistance bands, or weight machines. Resistance training is great for building muscles, maintaining flexibility and balance, increasing bone density, and even improving posture. It's essential as we age to maintain muscle size and support bone health because both are very hard to get back. The benefits for the brain include increased neurogenesis, which helps grow the brain and prevent degenerative diseases.

It's important to note that any type of exercise is better than no exercise. When trying to incorporate a new exercise, it's imperative you choose something sustainable. By participating in exercises you enjoy, you'll feel more motivated and excited at the prospect of working out. Not only will you reap the many physical benefits of exercise, but your brain health will also improve significantly. If you're unsure where to start, plenty of free resources are available online that can help you get your body moving. Finding quick workout videos or simply taking a brisk walk around the neighborhood is enough to get your blood pumping so that you can reap the endless benefits of exercise.

Turning Any Exercise into a Brain Exercise

What if you could make small adjustments that would provide an extra boost to your brain? The brain doesn't like ideal scenarios, as it finds those boring, so mixing it up is key.

Tips to make any exercise a brain-based exercise:

- Use a balance pad when doing a lunge, for example. Using an uneven surface not only challenges your muscles, but it also stimulates your brain.
- Sit on a balance/yoga ball when doing biceps curls or triceps extensions.
- Stand with one foot in front of the other when working your biceps or triceps.
- Do push-ups with your hands on a foam pad or a pillow.

How Much Exercise?

With all this knowledge about the incredible benefits of exercise on not only our physical health but also our mental and brain health, you must be wondering how much exercise you need to do in order to reap all these benefits. Most studies suggest that adults should aim for anywhere from ninety to 150 minutes of physical exercise per week, which works out to be thirty minutes of exercise, three to five times per week. Some studies claim that the biggest boost in brain health is linked to exercise sessions of forty-five to sixty minutes.

In all honesty, however, if you're looking to improve your brain health, including some sort of exercise is better than not doing any exercise at all. Be reasonable. Uprooting your entire routine and making unrealistic goals will likely cause you to feel overwhelmed and could, unfortunately, set you up for failure. It's better to start and complete five minutes of exercise than to plan for an hour, only to decide you don't have enough time and perform none.

To start, you could try incorporating just ten minutes a day: take a walk around the block or use the stairs at work instead of the elevator. As you develop a habit of exercising, you can increase the time and frequency of your workouts. Set yourself up for success, and remember that small changes are better than no changes.

For those with brain injuries, shorter spans of exercise, such as five minutes performed three to five times a day, are more beneficial and less likely to increase symptoms, as compared to doing all the exercise at once. Even if you don't have a brain injury, it's better to be active at multiple points throughout the day than only one thirty-minute window.

By following these tips, you'll find in no time that you're reducing your stress levels, feelings of anxiety, and brain fog; that you're improving your energy levels and memory, your ability to focus and process emotions; and that you're inadvertently slowing the brain-aging process and preventing the onset of brain diseases.

The evidence supporting the importance of exercise for brain health is indisputable. We can save our brains from incurable diseases and change our lives for the better if we exercise regularly. By taking matters into our own hands, we can improve our quality of life for the long haul and live longer, more fulfilling lives. Take a step back from all life's distractions, and think back to a simpler time. You'll find that you can learn a lot from how our ancestors lived, and by taking inspiration from them, you can live a healthy, happy life.

Summary

- Exercise has always been and will always be one of the best things we can do for our health.
- Nothing can replace the benefits of exercise.
- Find something you enjoy doing for exercise, as that will make it easiest.
- Any exercise is better than none; be consistent, and don't beat yourself up when there's a bump in the road.

"

By increasing cognitive flexibility,
we can quickly learn and apply
new information, problem solve in
innovative ways, and easily adjust
to changing conditions.

"

CHAPTER 8
Cognitive Exercises

As we go through our daily routines, we don't often consider all our bodies' processes that enable us to perform our daily tasks. Making coffee, eating breakfast, brushing our teeth, sending a text, or having a conversation—these things are all very routine. However, without a healthy brain, these mundane tasks that we take for granted might not be so simple. A healthy brain can process quickly and accurately while being flexible, traits that enable us to function as we do in our day-to-day lives. Any deviance from what's considered healthy can be very detrimental to what we know as normal. Throughout this chapter, we'll discuss cognitive flexibility, maintaining a healthy brain, how cognitive exercises affect the brain, and, of course, the various types of cognitive exercises.

Cognitive Flexibility

So what exactly is meant by "cognitive flexibility," and why is it so important?

First, let's paint a picture of what cognitive flexibility isn't. Imagine a three-year-old who has a daily routine governing when they eat, play, nap, and go to bed. What happens when this routine is thrown off schedule? Temper tantrums. This exemplifies the lack of cognitive flexibility that is found in a healthy, developed brain.

Cognitive flexibility refers to the brain's ability to adapt our behavior and thinking to best function in a situation. Often referred to as executive function, it's essentially our ability to react to new, changing, or unplanned events. It's our ability to change our behavioral response depending on the context of a situation. It can be considered a skill that allows us to analyze a new situation and generate a unique, appropriate response in order to achieve our goal.

Cognitive flexibility is important because it enables us to adapt to the constant changes in our daily lives. Without this flexibility, we'd be unable to switch from one situation to another. By increasing cognitive flexibility, we can quickly learn and apply new information, problem solve in innovative ways, and easily adjust to changing conditions. This can be advantageous in many aspects of our lives and can be demonstrated in our ability to follow directions, handle emotions, focus, and learn on the fly.

To better understand cognitive flexibility, let's consider this example: You're on your way to work, and you encounter a car accident that's causing a bunch of traffic that may result in you being late. You have two options. You can either sit in traffic and keep on the same route as usual or quickly figure out how to take the side streets and detour so that you can make it to work on time. Someone who is cognitively flexible would find an alternate route without much stress, quickly adapting to the situation. Alternatively, someone else would remain rigid and stick to their original route despite the delay and possibility of being late. Those who are more flexible can quickly adapt to this unexpected event and problem solve to find a solution.

People who suffer from brain disorders, be it ADHD or autism, typically lack cognitive flexibility. They easily perform routine activities; however, if their routine is disrupted, they may experience epic meltdowns. The same can be seen with adults who are cognitively declining or have dementia. Once these individuals become accustomed to a certain routine or patterned behavior, trying to adjust this routine can throw them for a loop, resulting in a breakdown of behavior, confusion, and memory impairment. This happens not only to those with developmental disorders or degenerative conditions; we also see these kinds of behaviors (to different degrees) in those who have suffered strokes, concussions, and traumatic brain injuries.

Setting the Brain Up for Success

Before we consider cognitive exercises, we should evaluate anything that may be affecting our brain health right now. Issues such as sleep apnea and deteriorating eyesight and hearing can negatively affect our brain health, despite requiring fairly simple fixes. Oftentimes, people can be stubborn, not wanting to give into these issues, but neglecting them can cause the brain to deteriorate.

We previously discussed sleep apnea in chapter 6, but it's important to repeat that you need to seek help if you suffer from it, as it impacts every aspect of your health, from weight and cardiovascular disease to brain health.

As we age, it's normal for our eyesight and hearing to start to slowly deteriorate. Once again, we can easily manage these issues. Wearing glasses or hearing aids or having cataract surgery can tremendously increase our quality of life. Being able to see and hear properly is essential to many aspects of our lives. However, not being able to see and hear can have awful effects on the brain. When our vision or hearing is impaired, certain parts of the brain don't get adequate input. As the input to these parts of the brain decreases, these areas slowly start to shrink.

We've already learned that the brain requires oxygen and nutrients to remain healthy. It also requires stimulation. Imagine trying to get strong by eating right, but never performing resistance exercises. You wouldn't actually get stronger. The same thing is true for the brain.

Providing input to the brain is essential to the health of the brain. Parts of the brain that lack proper input will ultimately shrink as we age, or not develop when we're young.

The better and stronger the input is into the brain, the greater the likelihood that the areas receiving and processing the input will stay healthy longer. Anything that we can do now to keep our brains healthy is of utmost importance, especially considering that addressing these issues now could slow down any dementia that might already be in the works. Remember, dementia usually starts ten to twenty years before a diagnosis is even made. For this reason alone, we should do everything in our power to keep our brains healthy and thriving. Besides dementia, cognitive stimulation and exercise are essential for those who have autism and those who have suffered brain injuries and strokes.

Effects of Cognitive Exercise on the Brain

We already know that keeping our brains healthy is incredibly important. This means we need to keep our brains flexible. Pretty much everything we do stimulates some sort of brain activity, whether washing the dishes, watching TV, or even reading this book right now. However, not all activities will stimulate all parts of the brain, and when we don't use certain parts of the brain, that part will start to shrink due to inactivity. As mentioned previously, the brain will recognize the parts that aren't getting any input, deem them unnecessary, and cause them to shrink as a result.

Cognitive exercises are beneficial to the brain because they can help build up parts of the brain that may not be used in average daily activities. By implementing cognitive exercise, we increase blood flow to certain areas of the brain and ameliorate cognitive flexibility. When performing any tasks, the brain often looks for the path of least resistance and utilizes existing, familiar nerve pathways as often as possible.

Have you ever driven home from work, parked in the driveway, and realized that you're not sure how you made it home? You remember absolutely no details of the drive. This is the perfect example of your brain working on autopilot. For activities like this, very little thought is required. It's easy to fall into routines as we perform the same tasks day in and day out. To stimulate the brain, we need to purposefully find activities that do so.

When we perform cognitive exercises, we stimulate different parts of the brain—parts that may not receive a lot of input in our daily lives. Activating these various parts of the brain increases blood supply, providing the brain cells with more oxygen and nutrients. The brain cells respond to this increase in blood flow by branching off to create new pathways in the brain, further generating more activity.

Just as we have physical goals when we work out, our goal when practicing cognitive exercises is to build strength and resilience in our brains, ultimately resulting in improved memory, attention, reasoning, planning, judgment, learning, and overall executive function. Cognitive exercise is any activity that challenges the brain to adapt and improve cognitive function. We want to find activities that require new and spontaneous thought, rather than routine thought. These activities will stimulate the brain through new experiences and enable our brain to grow and develop, rather than remain stagnant and shrink.

Ultimately, our brains are meant to keep us alive in the moment, but they are willing to sacrifice long-term health. Our brains will look for the simplest solution to resist expending too much energy. When faced with a new situation, the brain looks to past experiences to provide a similar, familiar solution. In order to work the brain, we need to participate in deliberate brain exercises—specifically targeting those areas that we struggle with. Practicing cognitive exercises will improve short-term memory as well as our visual, auditory, and spatial systems.

Types of Cognitive Exercise

In the same way that we require physical exercise to maintain our health, our brain needs cognitive exercise to remain healthy or to manage disease and disorders. Because it's important to focus on training the weakest parts of the brain, the type of exercise that's best for the brain will vary per individual. Think about when you're physically working out. If you discover that your left biceps isn't as strong as your right, you'd never simply ignore the left side. Instead, you'd focus on repetition and form in order to get the left side up to par with your right biceps.

The same goes for the brain. The parts of the brain that struggle the most are the parts that we should focus on. It may seem easier to ignore the parts of the brain that are impaired, but this would be detrimental to the brain's overall health.

In the last chapter, we discussed the benefits of physical exercise on the brain, some of which were mental clarity and focus. These benefits could be used to our advantage. Those who notice an increase in brain function after physical exercise could benefit from doing cognitive exercises immediately after their workout. The clarity and focus gained from physical exercise may enable some individuals to excel and better perform their cognitive exercise, making the exercises more effective in providing benefits to the brain.

Now, the type of exercise needed depends on the individual. There are a couple of exercises that improve brain function. The first example is an activity that uses flashcards with letters or numbers—the type that would be used to teach a child their letters and numbers. The activity requires the individual to shuffle the deck of cards and then sort them by placing the letters on the left and the numbers on the right. Alternatively, they could sort the letters A through M on the left and N through Z on the right. Any pattern of sorting these cards could work. This is an introductory, basic-level activity.

To bring it up a notch, we could try sorting while placing one foot in front of the other, and to progress even further, we could add in a rule that every time someone claps, you must change your arrangement. This means that whatever letters were being put to the left must now go to the right, and vice versa. This is called a pattern interrupt—a technique that disrupts a routine or behavioral pattern, to keep you on your toes, and challenges cognitive flexibility. When this activity with its progressions can be done quickly and accurately, we have a good indication of a healthier brain. If the individual participating in this activity has to pause to think about the change in pattern or struggles adapting, it's a sign that the brain isn't as healthy as it should be, which means they should keep practicing. Just as with physical exercise, repetition is key when it comes to improving brain health.

Our eyes are not only windows into the soul, but they are also windows into the health of our brain. When our eyes aren't functioning properly, it becomes hard to focus, concentrate, and even create memories. Think about having a conversation with someone. When they can maintain eye contact, we assume they're effectively listening and processing what we're telling them. Since the eyes are such a great indicator of brain health, another activity to try would be eye-movement-based therapy. An example of this is an exercise that involves placing a dot on a wall and standing about an arm's length away. Look at the dot and slowly move your head left and right about two inches in each direction. If the dot becomes blurry after doing this a couple of times, it's an indication that you're having issues and would benefit from a more in-depth evaluation.

[Disclaimer: Eye-movement exercises shouldn't be performed without expert help if the person doing the exercise suffers from autism, a brain injury, dementia, or has had a stroke, as many will perform it wrong and make themselves worse.]

Simple Exercises for the Brain

Activities you might consider to exercise your brain are:

- Jigsaw puzzles
- Sudoku
- Card games
- Reading
- Learning or teaching a new skill
- Learning an instrument
- Learning a new language

These activities can activate areas of the brain by challenging us in ways we don't experience on a regular basis. It's even been shown that playing some types of video games can lead to improvements in attention, problem-solving, and cognitive flexibility. However, we need to be careful with these more traditional activities. If we don't consistently increase the difficulty, the brain will eventually become accustomed to some of these puzzles and find ways to automate these activities. The brain will adopt routines and strategies for solving these problems, and they will no longer be challenging, which no longer provides important stimulation to the brain.

We're also looking for activities that are challenging and require coordination, keeping in mind that we want to get the most out of our exercises. Just like weight lifting, if you continuously do five-pound biceps curls and never progress to heavier weights, you probably won't see much progression in muscle strength, tone, or size. When working our arms, we consider more than just the biceps. To get a well-defined, muscular-looking arm, we need to work our biceps, triceps, and even our shoulders. We diversify our workout. The same should be done for the brain. We should diversify our cognitive training, activating several parts of the brain to increase flexibility and function.

Each individual needs to cater to their own cognitive goals. Cognitive exercise will look different depending on your own individual needs and cognitive impairments. Someone trying to manage dyslexia will participate in different activities than someone recovering from a brain injury. You need to find what works for you. Constantly assess your progress and adapt your training accordingly. This is best done by undergoing specific testing to evaluate the health of your brain, which we'll discuss in future chapters.

Summary

- Our brain can continue to learn and get stronger.

- Healthy brains have three things in common: speed, accuracy, and flexibility.

- Any activity that challenges the brain can be a form of brain-based stimulation: card games, board games, sudoku, and even activities like Ping-Pong.

- Specific testing can be done to evaluate the health of the brain in order to formulate a more individualized treatment plan.

While you may not always consider the consequences of events like these to be PTSD, they are forms of emotional trauma that create self-limiting beliefs that prevent us from reaching our potential.

CHAPTER 9
PTSD and Emotional Trauma

This chapter is one of the most important in the book. Over my years as a provider, I've seen PTSD and emotional trauma dictate whether someone improves or not with care.

There are a lot of preconceived notions about what causes PTSD. We judge others based upon our own experiences in life, but this approach misses the boat.

Let's compare developing PTSD to catching the flu. You can have one hundred people in a room where the flu virus is present, yet only a small percentage of those in the room will come down with the flu, depending on the strength of their immune system. The same is true with PTSD; many can be exposed to the same event, and each person will walk away from it differently. Some will have no issues at all, while it will forever change the lives of others.

Whether someone develops PTSD or not largely depends on the health of their brain, not the event itself. Keep this in mind as we work through this chapter.

What Is PTSD?

PTSD is considered a mental health condition triggered by a traumatic event, either being a witness to said event or actually experiencing it. You might think a traumatic event has to be a gruesome experience—sexual violence, physical abuse, military trauma, or witnessing a murder.

While all these events can trigger the disorder, PTSD can also present itself after an event that might be considered minor, even though the result is equally traumatizing. The events that result in trauma can be individual events, like a car accident, or ongoing events, such as emotional abuse. Those who suffer from PTSD may experience, among other symptoms, flashbacks, nightmares, severe anxiety, dissociation, and changes in mood.

Many different scenarios can cause PTSD or emotional trauma. First, we have to allow ourselves to recognize that trauma has occurred. This is where people often compare themselves to others, perhaps diminishing the experience they've had. They often rationalize it, trying to convince themselves that the event wasn't that bad. We need to forget this kind of mindset. We need to realize that we're allowed to have feelings, no matter how severe they may seem, based on events that have occurred.

This can look different for everyone. Maybe someone has been through a terrible divorce and now has issues with trusting others. Maybe someone else lacks self-worth because every time they asked their parents for something, the answer was always no. We can even see individuals who think they aren't good at anything because they were never complimented growing up. While you may not always consider the consequences of events like these to be PTSD, they are forms of emotional trauma that create self-limiting beliefs that prevent us from reaching our potential.

Of course, there's a scale to this. An event that triggers PTSD or emotional trauma for one individual may not trigger it in another. I've seen this time and time again, and I've learned to listen and not judge the experience, but to understand how the experience has shaped their life.

This is why it's imperative that we not compare experiences. We can't assume that someone's experience wasn't bad enough to warrant where they're landing mentally. We need to allow ourselves and others the grace to deal with their experiences in their own way. For example, after a car accident, some people have no issue getting behind the wheel right away, while others may have anxiety every single time they get in the car. This can really affect someone's quality of life; it can get to the point that they're unable to drive on the highway, while others may never be able to drive during inclement weather.

We can assess if we're experiencing PTSD or emotional trauma by evaluating how we react to a stressful event. If you notice that your symptoms flare with the event—increased brain fog, change in focus and concentration, dizziness, headaches—this is a clear PTSD response. This can also be seen in those with autoimmune disorders; if their disease symptoms flare when they're stressed, this may be a PTSD response.

PTSD and the Brain

As with everything else we've covered in previous chapters, PTSD affects the brain, which is an incredible organ. The brain has a mechanism in place—the amygdala—that acts as an alarm system. This primitive region of the brain drives our fight-or-flight response.

For our ancestors, our fight-or-flight response was essential for survival. Imagine getting too close to a bear, and it attacks you; you want to remember that experience so that you don't do it again. The amygdala is responsible for this association and response.

These days, the amygdala is triggered by simpler stressors that provoke emotions such as fear, anger, or anxiety. These stressors may be from driving, watching the news, social interactions, eating bad food, and many other activities or events. Regardless, the purpose of the amygdala is to notify you of danger at the right time and for the right reason, essentially to keep you safe. With individuals who suffer from PTSD, their amygdala no longer does its job correctly. This means that their fight-or-flight response can be triggered by something as simple as a firecracker or a car's backfire.

PTSD can also affect the prefrontal cortex, which we've learned is responsible for our executive function, which controls our emotions and focus. When working optimally, this region of the brain should be able to discern if what we're fearing is actually a threat that deserves our attention. It helps regulate the emotional responses triggered by the amygdala. When someone suffers from PTSD, the prefrontal cortex isn't always able to filter these threats, and it can give into the triggers brought on by the amygdala.

With the prefrontal cortex unable to effectively filter the amygdala's signals, those with PTSD will experience what may seem like extreme reactions to not-so-extreme stimuli. Those with PTSD may feel anxious around anything related to their trauma. They may also have strong physical reactions to situations that shouldn't provoke fear, and they'll often avoid situations that they think will trigger an intense emotional response or reaction. For example, based on their trauma, they might not be able to deal with hearing people raise their voices; because of this, they'll avoid confrontation with others at all costs to avoid the risk of triggering their PTSD response. Just the idea of someone raising their voice might stop them from having an important conversation because the emotional whirlwind that comes with being triggered isn't worth expressing their true thoughts and feelings.

Because PTSD is linked to the health of the brain, it's understandable that someone's age or health may influence what triggers PTSD. We know five-year-olds aren't the most rational human beings, so why would we expect trauma from that time to be rational?

Treating PTSD and Emotional Trauma

We now know that it's important to recognize and acknowledge PTSD or emotional trauma. Realizing there's an issue to be addressed is the first step in getting treatment. Leaving PTSD untreated can have negative effects on an individual's quality of life.

They may notice issues in their social relationships and in their ability to go about their normal daily tasks. Seeking treatment is essential to getting their life back on track.

To really understand the importance of addressing and treating PTSD, we can look at a study that was done on a group of individuals in their twenties. Researchers looked at people whose parents divorced when they were between the ages of four and six. What they found was that those whose parents divorced during that period of time were more likely to suffer from depression in their twenties than those who didn't experience their parents going through a divorce. There's also research linking severe PTSD during our forties with an increased risk of dementia.

We've learned in previous chapters that depression and anxiety can contribute to an unhealthy brain, which can lead to dementia and other types of cognitive decline. In order to avoid this decline's exacerbation by PTSD, we need to deal with it head-on.

Individuals commonly seek psychotherapy for PTSD and emotional trauma, and a therapist can treat these disorders in several ways. We often see patients undergo cognitive therapy, exposure therapy, or eye-movement desensitization and reprocessing. Alternatively, when these more traditional approaches are ineffective, patients may benefit from ketamine-based therapy or transcranial magnetic stimulation therapy. We'll discuss the effects of each type of treatment below:

- **Cognitive therapy**: This is a type of talk therapy, the goal of which is to help a patient identify the negative thoughts surrounding their trauma and try to modify their behaviors and thought patterns. Through this, patients can safely face their trauma and learn to cope with their fears and triggers effectively. With PTSD, this therapy is typically used alongside exposure therapy.

- **Exposure therapy**: This therapy will confront a patient, guided by a therapist, with a situation that's causing them fear. The goal here is to help the patient overcome the fear or anxiety surrounding a situation through consistent exposure to it, showing them that there's nothing to fear.

- **Eye-movement desensitization and reprocessing**: Similar to exposure therapy, this therapy confronts patients with their trauma, along with a series of guided eye movements that help them process their traumatic memories and change how they react to them.

- **Ketamine-based therapy**: Through ketamine infusions, we can modulate the heightened response in the brain, as well as change its processing of past events. With this therapy, patients don't have to talk about their experiences.

- **Transcranial magnetic stimulation therapy**: This is a noninvasive therapy that delivers repetitive magnetic pulses to the brain to stimulate nerve cells in the brain and reduce the symptoms of PTSD.

- **Psychedelics:** This is an ever-growing area of research. While it isn't being routinely used today, I believe it will be shortly. Therapies with substances such as psilocybin, MDMA, and others are showing great potential.

For those who have PTSD and brain injury, it's essential to have proper treatment for the injury and to rehabilitate the brain to the highest level. I rarely see brain injury patients who achieve the best results for their PTSD if they only go after the PTSD.

When an individual has suffered PTSD or emotional trauma, we can see a change in the brain, which shows a more heightened response. When considering the most effective treatments to mitigate this heightened response, ketamine-based therapy and transcranial magnetic stimulation therapy are my preferred methods because by the time someone comes to me, they've already tried the other options, which have failed. I think these methods work better, in part, because they don't require patients to revisit their trauma. By the time a patient accesses these types of treatment, they've been through years of therapy with insignificant success and are often very frustrated by always having to talk about their traumas. Their frustrations can create an unpleasant experience for them and hinder their ability to get to the deeper levels of therapy needed for recovery.

In addition, individuals can access many tools at home—simple things that can be incorporated into our daily lives to help improve our headspace. To start, there are plenty of motivational videos at our disposal online. Watching or listening to these kinds of videos, even if just for ten minutes in the morning, can help get us in the right mindset. By consistently listening to motivational clips, we can change our mindset to a more positive one.

Another at-home practice that's easy to incorporate is positive affirmation. Grab a dry-erase marker or lipstick and write something encouraging on your mirror—"You can do this!" or "You're awesome!" Look at yourself in the mirror and read these affirmations aloud to yourself multiple times a day. What we're doing here is basically what we call "Fake it till you make it." The more we instill positivity in our brains, the more we change the wiring and start to believe it and live it. Even if you don't believe it just yet, with consistent repetition, your brain will start to believe it.

Another activity you could try is to write down on a piece of paper one positive thing about yourself and your reason for moving forward. Do this every day. Come up with something new every single day and read back what you wrote the previous day. As time goes on, you'll have built a collection of positive feedback and reinforcement memos to yourself. The more notes you have to read, the more you'll be able to reinforce a positive mindset, acknowledge all the things you're grateful for, and realize that you're worth it and have what it takes to move forward.

The most important thing you can do when seeking help is to show up for yourself. You need to realize that you're worthy and deserve the best. Just as with working out or eating healthy, we see the biggest results when we're consistent. The same goes for therapy. Some of these activities are so incredibly simple that they take just a few minutes out of our day, but sometimes the simplest things are the hardest things to do. Consider buying or building a house: oftentimes people are so caught up in the details—the granite countertops and the tiles, for example. But if the foundation and framework aren't right, we can't house any of these beautiful fixtures.

The same applies to therapy. If we neglect to build the proper foundation through consistency, the fancier ketamine-based therapies or transcranial magnetic stimulation can't work to their full potential. Those who have the longest-lasting results build momentum through consistency, getting the most out of their recovery.

Create the Right Environment

While therapy is incredibly important when it comes to recovery, we also need to set up our environment for success. This starts with making sure you're surrounding yourself with the best support system you can. Healing from trauma is very difficult, if not nearly impossible, if you keep going back to the same toxic environment. This could mean that you have to cut off friends you've known for years or set firm boundaries in your relationships. They say that doing the same thing over and over and expecting different results is the definition of insanity. So if you enroll in therapy but still surround yourself with the same environment, you're essentially expecting a different result without making significant changes—something that's unlikely to happen.

Consider the rule of five. If, for example, our income is the average of the five people we spend the most time with, we can apply this same logic to our physical and mental health. This means that if the people we spend the most time with are consistently negative and bring us down, we need to remove them from our circle. If you have negative people in your top five, they need to go if you expect a better future. We can't allow others to bring us down and occupy our space in a negative way. We need to make room for positivity and surround ourselves with people who share the same mindset so that we can all thrive together.

Assess your work environment. Do you enjoy going to work? Do you like your coworkers? We spend so much time at work throughout the week that if the answer to these questions is anything other than yes, you need to take the time to really evaluate your situation. Obviously, quitting your job on the spot isn't advised. But if you're spending up to forty hours at work every week and not really enjoying yourself, it will be hard to implement the practices discussed above. We want to foster a positive environment to heal, and for some this might mean finding a new career path.

Another great thing we can do to help in recovery is to take vacations. In order to really recover, we need to separate ourselves from the everyday hustle and bustle of life. I'm sure we can all relate to how busy and stressful our daily lives can be. Now imagine trying to focus on yourself and your recovery in the midst of an already hectic life. It's difficult to truly commit to recovery when your focus is simply trying to survive the day or the week. Allow yourself the serenity of peace and quiet. For some, this might look like a camping trip, whereas for others it could be a beach getaway. Whatever brings you the most peace and serenity, do it. Disconnect from the world and connect to yourself. Give yourself permission to take this time to really heal and recover.

I can't stress enough the importance of recognizing and treating PTSD and emotional trauma. Allowing these traumas to affect you long term can be detrimental to your mental health and has the potential to cause greater problems for the brain if left untreated. Taking time every day to refocus our energy and really prioritize recovery and healing can make a tremendous difference, even if that means just incorporating very small and simple changes on a daily basis—being consistent will ensure success. It's important to realize that everyone has a different life experience and that everyone will react differently to certain events. Just because something seems very normal or familiar because it's what we've always known and grown up with, that doesn't mean it's optimal. We need to focus on what's optimal, and not what's common, in order to give ourselves the opportunity to heal.

Ultimately, we want to emphasize that, just because situations seem normal or common and everyone experiences stress, we cannot minimize the effects our experiences have on our mental health. It's okay to reach out for help and put yourself and your mental health first. Everything we experience impacts our lives, but how we choose to live impacts our brain health. In order to give our brains the best chance to be healthy as we age, we have to take care of ourselves.

Summary

- PTSD is a common problem that many experience.

- What causes PTSD for one person may not impact someone else.

- Whether or not PTSD develops largely depends upon how healthy the brain is.

- Many therapies can be utilized for PTSD, and there has been significant improvement in these regimens over the past few years.

- Everything you do is a signal to the brain. Send positive signals by getting your top five and doing things you enjoy.

"

Since the parts of our bodies are so interconnected, discovering any type of ailment or deficiency can affect many other different parts of our bodies, including the brain.

"

CHAPTER 10
Utilizing a Comprehensive Approach

Our bodies are incredible entities that require so many individual moving parts to function at an optimal level. What makes our bodies so fascinating is that everything is intertwined. For us to move our fingers to type words onto a page, so many different things are happening at the same time. The fact that the neurons in our brains can activate neurons in our spinal cords, which then activate the muscles in our arms and hands to do something so specific as hitting the right key on the keyboard almost every single time, is outstanding. In addition, while we perform our daily, mindless tasks, our bodies have to make sure we're breathing, our heart's pumping, and all our organs are performing the tasks essential to our survival. For this reason, it's important to make sure our brains are functioning as optimally as possible.

In the previous chapters, we learned many ways that we can drastically improve our brain health. By making changes to our lifestyle, we can set our brains up for future success. Doing everything in our power to maintain our brain health as we age is exceptionally important, especially when it comes to degenerative brain diseases. We're well aware now of the factors—inflammation, energy crisis, impaired connectivity, injury, and issues with blood flow and oxygen—that affect our brain health. Managing these issues is paramount when it comes to supporting and maintaining our brain health. Throughout this chapter, we're going to explore how looking at and analyzing lab work can influence these core factors that contribute to the health of our brains.

Why Look at Lab Work?

When considering our general health, performing routine blood work seems like a no-brainer. Our family physician will generally send us for blood work during our annual physical to make sure our bodies are functioning as they should. Typically, routine blood work is used as part of preventive health care, but it can also be used to diagnose certain illnesses. Doctors can measure cholesterol levels and our risk of developing cardiovascular disease, among many other ailments.

In addition to blood work, doctors can analyze saliva, stool, or urine samples. These types of lab tests can tell us so much about what's going on in our bodies and can empower us to make informed decisions about our bodies and our health. Knowledge is power, and the more we know about what's going on in our bodies, the better we can care for them.

Since the parts of our bodies are so interconnected, discovering any type of ailment or deficiency can affect many other different parts of our bodies, including the brain. Any ailment or disease may have some effect on the brain, even if it's not considered a brain disease. The lab tests that can be performed and the markers being examined, while not fully comprehensive, can provide a great starting point for considering what may be happening in the brain.

Let's think about the brain as a plant for a moment. For a plant to grow and thrive, it needs to have adequate water, the right balance of nutrients within the soil, the right amount of sunlight, and the perfect environmental elements. The same can be said about the brain. To foster the right environment for a healthy brain, we must first examine all the appropriate lab markers. The lab tests we want to consider when it comes to the brain are blood, saliva, and urine.

Blood Work

At some point in our lives, surely we've all had to get blood work done for one reason or another: a routine checkup or a proactive test to rule out ailments that run in the family, or maybe we're just feeling lethargic and want to find out if there's an underlying issue. There's so much we can learn about our health through analyzing blood work.

The first thing we would like to consider is the CBC panel—a complete blood count. This test is an essential starting point to evaluate our overall health by assessing white and red blood cells, hemoglobin, hematocrit, and platelets. With this, we can detect many different disorders such as anemia, the presence of infection, nutritional deficiencies, bone-marrow problems, or even cancer.

With blood work, we can also do what's called a comprehensive metabolic panel. This test can measure glucose, minerals, electrolytes, blood-protein levels, and the health of our liver and kidneys. If any of these are off, it will surely affect our brain health. These are the basics, but they're such a small part of the picture that a deeper dive is needed to get answers.

Vitamins and Minerals

A low number of red blood cells may be due to low levels of iron or vitamin B, which can have a negative impact on the brain. This diagnosis could lead to cognitive dysfunction, neurological injury, and decreased levels of oxygen to the brain. For this reason, those with anemia may experience headaches, fatigue, dizziness, and brain fog as side effects.

It's also important to consider our level of vitamin D, which is crucial to helping regulate our immune system. Vitamin D deficiency has also been linked to a range of cognitive disorders as it's involved in regulating many genes that are crucial for brain function. Low levels of vitamin D are also routinely seen in those who have depression.

Another marker that should be examined is homocysteine, which is a measure of how well our bodies use vitamin B. Typically vitamin B breaks down homocysteine into other substances our bodies need. If we find high levels of homocysteine in the blood, this means that there could be a deficiency in vitamin B that's causing elevated levels of homocysteine. This elevated level of homocysteine is considered a risk factor for heart disease, stroke, and dementia. It's correlated with vascular inflammation, which is not only bad for the heart, but can also impact the flow of blood and oxygen throughout the body and, of course, the brain.

Homocysteine levels do not have to be lab high in order to be toxic for the brain. A range of eleven or greater is linked to dementia; some think the critical point should be lower than that.

Essential Fatty Acids

Essential fatty acids such as DHA and EPA are critically important for overall health, from our cardiovascular system to our brain. A blood test called OmegaCheck, or omega-3 index, will reveal your levels. This will measure total omegas, as well as an omega 06:03 ratio. The omega 06:03 ratio should be a 3 or 4; when it is higher, this indicates the presence of a lot of inflammation. In the United States, the total omega lab range is greater than 5.5, while in Japan the average individual is closer to 8. Low levels have the same impact on longevity, starting at the age of sixty-five, as smoking does. So, yes, it's a big deal to know this level and, if necessary, get it corrected.

Blood Sugar

When it comes to blood sugar, we want to look a little deeper. We want to first consider our fasting insulin. When our fasting insulin levels are higher than the optimal range of 4 to 8, this could mean that we're developing insulin resistance. This doesn't need to be lab high to be an issue.

Another way to look at insulin is to look at a marker called C-peptide. This will give us an idea of what's happening with our insulin. C-peptide is released from the pancreas at the same rate as insulin; therefore, it's a good measure to check whether we're releasing insulin at adequate levels. Insulin resistance is not only harmful in that it could be a sign you're developing diabetes, but it also affects the brain.

Did you know that insulin resistance impacts the brain before the rest of the body, and it may manifest as brain fog, poor memory, and mood changes?

Insulin acts as a growth factor and plays a large role in how the brain connects. If we develop insulin resistance, we can't expect the brain to connect and repair in the way that it would if our insulin levels were normal. Additionally, a side effect of insulin resistance is inflammation, which can damage the brain and which also prevents the brain from having a steady energy supply—three things we've already learned contribute to an unhealthy brain. Leaving this unchecked can be very detrimental, not only to our overall health but also to our brain health.

While considering blood sugar and diabetes, we also often think of A1C levels. Typically the hemoglobin A1C test is used to diagnose prediabetes or type 2 diabetes. To break this down, we have to expand on how this test works. Essentially, hemoglobin is the part of the red blood cell that carries oxygen to our cells. Like oxygen, glucose is also able to bind to the hemoglobin in our cells through a process called glycosylation. The A1C test basically measures the level of glucose attached to our hemoglobin. When the level goes up, this creates inflammation. The danger of an elevated A1C, aside from diabetes, is that it affects the function of our red blood cells and damages them. That's why having diabetes or elevated blood sugar can cause such widespread issues.

In severe cases of diabetes, sometimes patients will experience neuropathy in their feet. If there's neuropathy in the feet, it's likely this could be happening in the brain as well, as there's not enough blood flow or oxygen reaching the brain to allow it to heal and repair in the most effective way. The effects of this can be magnified if someone is dealing with a brain injury, a developmental disorder, or a degenerative disorder. It can make recovery nearly impossible for these people.

Hormones

We've previously covered the importance of energy levels throughout the body. A great way to measure energy is to look at how our thyroid is functioning. The thyroid releases and controls our thyroid hormones, which are responsible for our metabolism. Our metabolism is the process by which food is converted to energy within the body. Generally, when they want to look at the function of the thyroid, most doctors test TSH and T3. However, sometimes simply taking thyroid medication may not be enough. To get a comprehensive look, we must also consider other markers of thyroid function, as well as autoimmune markers such as thyroglobulin antibodies and thyroid peroxidase antibodies. Other markers of thyroid function include T4, free T3, free T4, and reverse T3. The presence of these antibodies indicates an autoimmune response is happening in the thyroid, and the immune system is essentially attacking the normal, healthy thyroid tissue.

If the body is confused enough to start attacking the thyroid, how do we know other parts of the body are not being attacked? Some research shows that elevated levels of these antibodies could also impact the cerebellum, the part of the brain responsible for coordination. This happens as a result of molecular mimicry. Think of it this way: Have you ever seen someone from a distance, and they looked as if they were someone you know? Maybe they were the same height and had the same hair color and same build, but as you got closer and could make out the details of their face, you realized it wasn't the person you thought it was.

Well, when the brain and immune system are functioning properly, they should be able to make these same distinctions between foreign structures and those that occur naturally in the body. In the case of autoimmunity, our immune cells, due to their inability to differentiate these structures, start attacking the cells and tissues in our body as if they were a danger to us. This can cause all sorts of devastation in the human body, including inflammation, which is why it's imperative to get any autoimmune issues under control.

The last hormones we'll consider when it comes to blood work are testosterone, estrogen, progesterone, and cortisol. These hormones play an important role in how certain neurotransmitters, such as dopamine and serotonin, act. Furthermore, they can help with inflammation and with connections within the brain, which by now we all know are incredibly important in maintaining a healthy brain. So if these hormones are out of balance, they can be very detrimental to our brain health.

Saliva Test

A less common lab test is a saliva test. These tests are noninvasive and typically require you to collect a test tube of saliva to be sent off and analyzed in a lab.

As mentioned above, hormone levels are very important when it comes to both overall health and brain health. Female hormones (estradiol, progesterone, and testosterone) can be easily measured through a simple saliva test.

A lot of research has been done to examine what happens in the postmenopausal brain due to the decrease in hormones. Women often experience an array of side effects during menopause, including irritability, mood swings, and brain fog. Luckily, if we can quantify the level of hormones through a saliva test, we can manage the hormone levels. The preferred hormone replacement method is bioidentical hormone replacement therapy.

We can also look at cortisol levels through a saliva test. Produced by our adrenal glands, cortisol is typically at its highest level in the morning, gradually tapering down throughout the day. Our cortisol levels can be thrown off by many factors, including brain injuries, dementia, and even chronic stress. When our cortisol levels are off, this can impact our energy levels, create a chronic state of inflammation, and break down brain tissue. Increased cortisol levels due to stress will ultimately shrink the hippocampus, the part of the brain responsible for learning and memory. For this reason, it's important to check and manage our cortisol levels. (It's important to note that these levels can fluctuate day to day, so it's best to have a series of tests to figure out your average.)

Urine Analysis

Although blood and saliva tests are great ways to assess how well our bodies are functioning, other aspects of our health can't be evaluated through these measures. This is where we can utilize urine tests.

In reference to the brain, we want to first focus on what's called a urine environmental toxin test. Essentially, this test measures how many toxins we're removing (not the total amount of toxins in our body).

We're exposed to toxins every day through our food, water, personal care products, and the air. It's basically impossible to avoid taking in toxins, but knowing the level of our toxic burden is important.

As we're exposed to certain toxins, our body is unable to metabolize them, and they end up bioaccumulating in our bodies. However, the amount that accumulates in each individual's tissues will vary.

While we're growing and developing, these toxins and heavy metals accumulate in our bones. Eventually, when we start losing bone density as we age, these chemicals are released into our bloodstream and inevitably reach our brain. An excess burden of these toxins can cause developmental brain disorders and has even been seen in children with autism.

Even though many of the toxins for which we are being tested have been banned throughout the world, they're still found in cord blood decades later. This means that they're being passed down from our parents and are still in the environment because they last so long.

To go along with the urine environmental toxin test, a blood test called a Cyrex test, specifically array 11, can be done through a lab that will let us know what's happening from an immune perspective, rather than just the exposure level. By doing both this and the urine test, we can see the immune consequence and how much inflammation is being caused by our exposure to these toxins.

Most importantly, these toxins are very harmful to our mitochondria, which produce energy in our cells and, when disrupted, can shift our immune response and cause all sorts of issues in the body. This explains why many of these toxins were banned.

While we're unable to completely escape these toxins, knowing our level of exposure and our immune response will enable us to manage them or even try to remove those that we can.

Taking control of our overall health is very important. Any preexisting health conditions can greatly impact our brain. Oftentimes when something is off in our body, it affects several different areas of the body, even if it seems it can be treated easily through traditional medicine.

To address any underlying issues, we should consider starting with comprehensive blood work, a saliva test, and a urine test. From there, we should have a pretty good understanding of what's happening in our bodies and what might be keeping us from success. However, before we start spending money on fancier, more costly tests, we should address the issues found through the more basic tests, like diabetes or thyroid problems. If something like diabetes isn't being properly managed, it would be a waste of time and money to move on to other testing because, when left untreated, diabetes can wreak havoc on our entire system. Addressing and getting each issue under control and then reevaluating would be the most proactive way to get the brain on track for recovery.

Anything that throws off our energy production and utilization, causes inflammation, or impacts our vascular blood flow will affect our brain health. If these issues go untreated, it's nearly impossible to expect the brain to be able to develop or recover from diseases to its full potential. If the environment isn't right, the brain is being set up for failure. And despite investing time, money, and effort into recovery, you'll likely notice few to no results. We have to make sure we foster the right environment to give our brains the best chance for recovery.

Summary

- Labs build upon everything you've learned in this book so far.

- Knowing your vitamin, homocysteine, and omega levels is important to your health.

- Blood sugar and insulin levels not only impact the body but also the brain.

- Hormones impact health and affect much more than reproduction.

"

We can consider taking care of our brain in the same way that we think about exercising. There are many exercises that can be done at home, using only our body weight, but to really push our fitness to the next level, we may require more equipment, weights, and knowledge from a trainer.

"

CHAPTER 11
Evaluating and Strengthening the Brain

A s we begin this chapter, it's important to emphasize that discussing brain health is all-encompassing. The brain can't be examined as a freestanding entity. When treating the brain, we must treat the entire person, the whole body. What happens in one part of the body has the ability to affect the entire body.

Surely you've heard the saying "If it's not broken, don't fix it," but when it comes to the body, we can't always visually see that it's broken. Remember, our body will compensate to keep us functional in the moment, but it will sacrifice the future. We need to identify and correct the compensations early to prevent diseases that take years to develop. As we've mentioned previously, Alzheimer's has been in the works for ten to twenty years by the time a diagnosis is made. We must look a little more in depth to find the issues that drive these processes.

Now, up to this point, we've examined the basic, foundational principles of improving brain and body health. In chapter 10, we discussed how labs should be considered and that they give us an overall idea of what's happening in the entire body on a deeper level, things that we can't see just by looking at someone. Examining labs is a great place to start.

We can consider taking care of our brain in the same way that we think about exercising. There are many exercises that can be done at home, using only our body weight, but to really push our fitness to the next level, we may require more equipment, weights, and knowledge from a trainer. By both exploring beyond what we already know and expanding our fitness routines outside our living rooms, we might be able to reach goals that would otherwise not be possible. The same can be said about our brains. Sometimes, in order to get the best results, we must seek help from a professional.

Throughout this chapter, we'll explore a variety of tools that may be used to improve brain health. These methods are all based around the concepts we've learned about what constitutes a healthy brain—energy, inflammation, connection, and blood and oxygen flow—and will provide further avenues we can explore for improving brain health.

Evaluating Brain Function

Eye Movement and Balance Testing

Oftentimes when we think about our eye health, we consider our vision. For example, do we need glasses? Or maybe we're experiencing some sort of degenerative disease like cataracts, glaucoma, or macular degeneration. While these issues should be examined and addressed, the eyes can tell us so much more about the brain.

You've probably heard the saying "The eyes are the windows to the soul," and while this may be true on a metaphoric level, on a realistic level, we can more accurately describe the eyes as windows to the brain. We can map out almost the entire brain just by examining eye movements.

In order to measure eye movement, it's recommended that you find a clinic that uses videonystagmography, also known as video-oculography. This test is performed by placing over the eyes special goggles that record and measure a variety of eye movements. While wearing the goggles, the patient watches moving dots on a TV screen. The dots, based upon the task, may be stationary or may move at different speeds and in different directions.

Most people believe that they know what's going on with their eyes because they have regular checkups with their optometrist and are correcting their vision with glasses. However, after completing and reviewing the results from a videonystagmography, nearly 80 percent of my patients are shocked to see what's actually happening with their eyes.

Typically, people don't notice the movements occurring in their eyes because the brain compensates for these movements to keep us stable. While the brain has this ability to compensate, that's not a sign the brain is healthy. So it's important to explore and find out if something is going on—the brain will work hard to keep things on track, even if it expends more energy to do so. This is one of the reasons why chronic fatigue and behavioral problems are so common when the brain isn't healthy.

Eventually, this compensation may break down, which can lead to an abundance of symptoms. Many people who have suffered from a concussion, TBI, or stroke will find it exceedingly hard to recover if this testing isn't done to identify the part of the brain that needs rehabilitation. Besides brain injuries, this is also great for dementia and neurodevelopmental conditions such as autism.

Along with the eye-movement tests, it's beneficial to simultaneously participate in balance testing, preferably using a computerized system that records your movements. This enables you to track your progress and quantitatively measure whether there's an improvement or not. Balance reflects our brain health and integrates information from our vision, vestibular, and proprioceptive systems. (Proprioception is information from joints and muscles such as the cervical spine and lower extremities.)

Quantitative Electroencephalogram Test

To further investigate what's happening in the brain, we can look at how the brain is connecting by using a quantitative electroencephalogram (qEEG) test, also referred to as brain mapping. This test can measure electrical activity in the form of brain-wave patterns. Think of this as the speed at which the brain communicates as it essentially breaks down what's happening in each brain wave. Brain waves reveal a lot of information relevant to our overall brain function, including stress levels, thought patterns, and emotions. The qEEG can identify brain-wave patterns that correlate with depression, anxiety, cognitive impairment, concussion, autism, and learning disabilities such as ADHD and dyslexia.

By identifying any deviations from a healthy brain, we can apply and streamline the appropriate treatments for each individual's unique needs. Treatment isn't a one-size-fits-all deal. What might help one person may not help another. By really digging deep and finding exactly where the issue is originating, we can personalize the perfect treatment. This will look slightly different for everyone, but it will be based on foundational principles that apply to every healthy brain.

Treatments

At this point, we've learned more ways to identify issues with the brain, which is incredibly important when it comes to finding the best treatment. There are many ways that we can go about treating the brain, and we've already explored many that can be done at home. We should focus on our diet, exercise, and brain exercises (among others) to jump-start brain health. While these are all great and should be incorporated into our daily lives to heal and recover, sometimes we have to call in a professional. There's only so much we can do on our own, and it's okay to seek help.

Neurofeedback

The first type of treatment we'll touch on is neurofeedback, a type of neurotherapy that relies on conditioning the brain to reinforce healthy brain function. You can think about it as being similar to the theory about Pavlov's dogs. We all know the story: every time Pavlov fed his dogs, he rang a bell. Finally, when the dogs heard the bell ringing, they automatically started salivating; they had made a connection between the sound of the bell and their meal. This was done so repetitively that if Pavlov rang the bell and there wasn't any food, the dogs still salivated.

The same principles can be applied to training the human brain. Once we pinpoint the areas of the brain that have deviated from what's considered normal, we can utilize neurofeedback to get things back on track. Neurofeedback works by retraining suboptimal brain waves to enable the brain to function to the best of its ability.

The therapy involves placing electrodes on the head to track brain-wave activity. The activity is then shown to the patient who is encouraged to change the activity level to one that's more desirable. Depending on the equipment that's used, the patient will hear sounds or see different visual cues to let them know their brain is doing what it should. This is done on more of a subconscious level. Eventually, the brain, craving this type of feedback, will act in a way that triggers the feedback (hence the name "neurofeedback"). The key here, as with all brain rehab, is repetition. The more we reward the brain for doing the right thing, the more the brain recognizes the reward and feels encouraged to act in a way to receive the reward.

Many symptoms and conditions see great improvement with this therapy. It's been utilized in treating a wide range of brain disorders, such as anxiety, depression, ADHD, autism, concussions, and even migraines. The key, as always, is repetition and reinforcing positive changes for the brain. The more we partake in neurofeedback, the stronger the new connections become, and we can truly heal the brain. This therapy has seen tremendous improvements over the past ten years, allowing for more accuracy and fewer sessions to see improvement.

As a result, this therapy has become increasingly popular, but I see the best results with children. Also, as noted before, I don't like to use it as a one-trick pony because, in doing so, the fail rate goes up.

Transcranial Magnetic Stimulation

This therapy is typically used for depression; however, there's been promising research that shows its benefits for other brain disorders. The patient will be given magnetic pulses that cause neurons to fire in a new pattern that can create new connections throughout the brain, changing the brain patterns that may be involved in depression or other brain diseases, and creating healthier connections.

Though these are still considered off-label uses for transcranial magnetic stimulation, it's been shown to be helpful in treating insomnia, anxiety, ADHD, concussions, and cognitive impairment. Currently, these uses are not all FDA approved; however, they're being used in other countries, and current research supports these off-label uses. In our clinic we see a lot of improvement with not only depression, but also focus, concentration, brain fog, and processing speed.

There's a lot of potential with these therapies, and even though they aren't approved right now, that doesn't mean they should be dismissed. We can achieve a lot with transcranial magnetic stimulation, especially when the research is translated into clinical practice. This is definitely a therapy we should keep an eye on.

Hyperbaric Oxygen Therapy

As we know, lack of oxygen flow to the brain is very harmful. With hyperbaric oxygen therapy, patients are placed in a closed chamber in which the atmospheric pressure is increased, raising the amount of oxygen that gets into the tissues. This can be done in a hard-shell or soft-shell chamber, with little to no difference in results in my experience. The goal with this therapy is to hyper-oxygenate the tissues, allowing them to perform more optimally, in turn setting the brain up for success.

There are other interesting uses for this therapy as well: it can help speed up the healing of carbon-monoxide poisoning, gangrene, and other infections in which tissues are starved for oxygen. It's routinely used in traditional medicine for wounds and gangrene not responding to regular care. Essentially, this therapy allows the body access to more oxygen than would be possible under normal air-pressure conditions.

This therapy on its own may be enough for some people, but for most it falls short if used as a one-trick pony. Most patients require a combination of a few types of therapy. Let's go back to the fitness comparison. In order to reach peak fitness level, we need to incorporate several aspects to our lifestyle: nutrition, exercise, and sleep. If one of these pillars is missing, we likely won't see the highest potential results. The same can be said for any therapy to support the brain. If you focus on only one type of therapy, you do yourself a disservice, especially if you're not satisfied with the results. I routinely see patients who have tried forty to sixty sessions without results because they weren't evaluated appropriately to see if they were a good fit. When you don't get desired results with this as a stand-alone therapy, it's a clear sign you should incorporate layers of therapy to stack the deck in your favor.

Eye Movement and Balance Therapy

We previously talked about how important eye movement and balance testing are when it comes to evaluating brain health. When testing identifies dysfunction, we use the results to create a customized plan for you. For example, specific eye-movement patterns may be used to strengthen connections in the brain. (As noted previously, we won't go into specific therapies because it's essential they're performed properly or they can make you worse.) Balance therapies are routinely used as well, but remember—don't perform these in isolation as results are best when layered together.

Nutritional Therapy

We previously talked about eating for a healthy brain, as well as adding some nutritional supplements to help with inflammation and brain health. These may include oral supplements and injectable vitamins, as well as peptides and amino-acid sequences that are naturally produced in the body and which can be found at specialty compounding pharmacies. Incorporating these into our routine can have profound impacts on the body overall, but more specifically will improve the brain's ability to heal, recover, and perform to its highest potential.

Finding Help

Now that you have the knowledge to seek out treatment, you're probably wondering where to start. Where can you find the treatment you're looking for? Because not many clinics have all these resources under one roof, you may have to visit a few different professionals to cover your bases.

A great place to start would be to seek out a clinic that does chiropractic neurology or functional neurology. These clinics would be equipped with a lot of these diagnostic tools, specifically the videonystagmography (eye-movement) and balance tests; some may perform the qEEG test as well.

What might be harder to find in the same clinic that offers these tests is the transcranial magnetic stimulation therapy and hyperbaric oxygen therapy. It's important to remember that just because you may not find all of these under the same roof, it doesn't mean they should be forgotten; not everything I've listed may be necessary for your unique case.

While I love chiropractic neurology, many of the clinics don't focus on immune health. You'll need to find another provider to address that if they don't.

Immunity and energy are the two biggest factors I see that determine long-term and not short-term results.

In order to have the best chance for recovery, we need to address all aspects. We don't want to put all our eggs in one basket and hope that the one therapy we choose will give us all the success we're seeking. People waste a lot of time and money by doing this. To really succeed, it's imperative to diversify the therapy being used. By incorporating several different types of therapy, we're investing in our health and setting ourselves up to win.

People will often try only one type of therapy and then bash it because it didn't work. We've learned throughout this book that our body is all-encompassing, that what happens in one part of the body affects another (seemingly unrelated) part of the body because our bodies are intertwined into one cohesive working unit. When we allow ourselves the opportunity to engage in different types of therapy that target different parts of the brain and body, we're allowing for a synergistic effect to provide greater results than any single therapy can provide on its own.

Overall, it should become more and more clear just how intertwined our system is. In order to really heal, it's imperative we identify the issues at hand and treat them accordingly. To keep our brains performing at their optimal capacity, we know that we have to reduce inflammation, address energy crises, improve connectivity, and maintain sufficient blood and oxygen flow. These are the main things that we know will cause the brain to become unhealthy.

Plenty of tests are available to examine exactly what's happening in the brain. By utilizing these tests, we can home in on repairing and reversing the damage. Being aware of exactly what's going on will enable professionals to find the best treatment made just for you. If the provider you've been using for a couple of years isn't doing the job, it's okay to move on and try a different approach. Don't stay in a place that isn't helping you.

By combining everything we've learned in this chapter, along with what we learned in previous chapters, we can build a really good foundation. We can not only address the basics of our health, but when we bring it all together with lab work and finding out how our brain is connecting, a wide range of brain ailments may be helped, starting with depression, concussion, dizziness, autism, memory loss, and brain injury.

Having the ability to know exactly what's happening through comprehensive evaluation is the most important factor in finding the appropriate treatment.

"

The Brain-Body Reset not only
improves the conditions that
have been weighing you down,
but it can also lift you to a new
level of health that you've never
experienced before.

"

CHAPTER 12
Want Individualized Guidance and Extra Help?

Congratulations on making it this far in your journey to better brain health. You've managed to do what most others will never do. You've invested in yourself and taken crucial steps toward improving the health of both your brain and your entire body.

Over the course of the past eleven chapters, you've taken a deep dive into the inner workings of your brain. Together we've learned about the symptoms of an unhealthy brain, the hazards of inflammation, how the brain uses energy, and how to fuel our bodies to feed our brain correctly. We've also delved into the importance of a good night's rest, why exercise is crucial to good brain health, and how certain mind games and activities can keep your brain healthy and strong for years to come.

Depending on your unique situation, you may have spent years struggling with some of the symptoms of an unhealthy brain, and if you're like most of us, you probably didn't even realize it. My hope for you is that you've managed to implement some of the foundational steps included in these pages and that you've found some relief and improvement in your overall well-being.

Fortunately, your quest for good health doesn't have to stop when this book does. Through years of hard work and dedication, I've created two specific programs that you can enroll in to help you continue along your path to achieving optimal brain health.

One-on-One Coaching

Located in the beautiful state of Idaho is my personal office. Many patients choose to travel here, where I can meet them in person and provide them with personalized care. Depending upon your individual needs, you may choose to stay for a day or even a few weeks. Some patients find that a two-week stay provides them with the intensive therapies they require to transform their health and obtain results that haven't been achievable through years of trying other methods.

During my one-on-one coaching program, I'll perform detailed lab work that will help me determine what issues are plaguing you and how I can help improve your overall health. By figuring out why you haven't been successful at getting better in the past, we'll be able to prevent further illness in the future.

My one-on-one sessions start with creating and executing a customized plan, identifying factors that will limit your results, and providing education on what's happening in your body and brain. I strive to give all my patients a complete, thorough understanding of their health and what needs to be done to improve it.

We'll look at the therapies that will best benefit you, and I'll create a care plan based on your unique set of symptoms and personal requirements. While we're together, we'll spend an extensive amount of time working on helping you achieve the best health possible. This is an intensive program designed to get you the results you need as quickly as possible.

If this sounds like the right method for you, contact my team and request a free help strategy session. We'll obtain all the information we require and will discuss your goals for the program. If we both decide that you're the right fit, we'll move forward and book an appointment.

The Brain-Body Reset

If one-on-one sessions aren't a good match for your specific requirements, we have another option that's helped countless others reach an improved level of brain health. The Brain-Body Reset is a ten-week program in which a guide will dive even deeper into the basics we've reviewed in this book, providing you a level of accountability to take your health to a new level.

Throughout the course, you'll be taught how to change your nutrition to positively impact your health. We'll look at sleep patterns, energy expenditure, and weight loss and give you simple yet effective techniques to implement what you're learning in your daily life.

At the end of this course, our patients often see a drastic transformation in how they feel. Not only are their symptoms significantly reduced, but they also feel younger and clearer and have an increased level of energy.

The Brain-Body Reset not only improves the conditions that have been weighing you down, but it can also lift you to a new level of health that you've never experienced before. We teach you how to harness your body and brain to achieve maximum wellness.

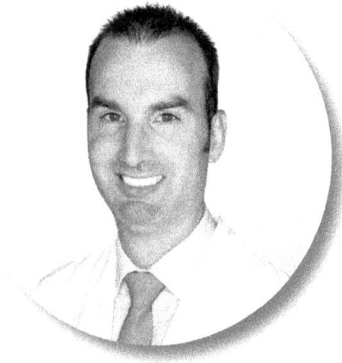

DOCTOR

Let's Connect

Find out more about Dr. Spencer Zimmerman
at the following links!

Official Website: DrSpencerZimmerman.com

Facebook: Dr. Spencer Zimmerman

YouTube: @dr.spencerzimmerman2256

Instagram: @drspencerzimmerman